Basic Introduction
to
Bioelectromagnetics

Basic Introduction
to
Bioelectromagnetics

Carl H. Durney
Douglas A. Christensen

CRC Press

Boca Raton London New York Washington, D.C.

147676

Library of Congress Cataloging-in-Publication Data

Durney, Carl H. 1931–
    Basic introduction to bioelectromagnetics / Carl H. Durney,
Douglas A. Christensen.
        p. cm.
    Includes bibliographical references and index.
    ISBN 0-8493-1198-5 (alk. paper)
    1. Electromagnetics--Physiological effect. 2. Electromagnetic
fields. I. Christensen, Douglas A. II. Title.
QP82.2E43D87 1999
612′.01442—dc21

for Library of Congress

99-29332
CIP

Preface

While doing research in bioelectromagnetics (the interaction of electromagnetic fields with biological systems) for more than 25 years, we have sensed the need that some life scientists have to understand the basic concepts and characteristic behaviors of electromagnetic (EM) fields so they can work effectively with physicists and electrical engineers in interdisciplinary research. Because most EM books are based heavily on vector calculus and partial-differential equations, however, little written information about EM fields satisfies this need. Many times over the years, life scientists have asked us for references to EM books appropriate for them, but we could give none. We have written this book in an effort to fulfill that need, as well as to help others who want to learn about electromagnetics but do not have the mathematical background to understand typical books on electromagnetics.

This book explains the basic concepts, fundamental principles, and characteristic behaviors of electric and magnetic fields to those who do not have a background in vector calculus and partial differential equations. In particular, it is intended for life scientists collaborating with engineers or physicists in work involving the interaction of electromagnetic fields with biological systems. It should also be helpful to health physicists, industrial hygienists, and public health workers concerned with possible hazards or beneficial applications of electromagnetic field exposure, and those concerned with magnetic resonance imaging, optical interactions with tissue, and wireless communication devices. In stark contrast to typical EM books that require a background in vector calculus and partial-differential equations, this book requires only a background in algebra (some acquaintance with trigonometric functions would also be helpful). It explains in detail the basic concepts, fundamental principles, and characteristic behaviors of EM fields. The explanations include a minimum of mathematical relationships with the emphasis on qualitative behaviors and graphical descriptions. Nevertheless, in spite of the de-emphasis on mathematics, the concepts of EM field theory are still treated comprehensively and accurately. The material covers the entire frequency spectrum from dc up through optical frequencies. Practical explanations are given to help readers understand real situations involving EM fields. One hundred and eighty-seven illustrations are included to augment qualitative explanations.

The first chapter introduces the fundamentals of EM field theory and explains how characteristic behaviors can be effectively grouped in three categories defined by the wavelength of the EM fields compared with the size of the objects with which they interact: (1) when the wavelength is much larger than the size of the objects, (2) when it is about the same, and (3) when the wavelength is much smaller than the size of the objects. Chapters 2, 3, and 4, respectively, explain the characteristic behaviors in each of these three categories. Chapter 5 explains some of the principles of EM dosimetry. The book concludes with Chapter 6, which gives a few examples of medical applications of EM fields to illustrate some of the principles discussed in earlier chapters. We sincerely hope that this book will be useful to intended readers. We welcome comments and suggestions for improving it.

Authors

Douglas A. Christensen was born in Bakersfield, CA December 14, 1939. He attended Brigham Young University in Provo, UT, graduating with a BSEE degree in electrical engineering in 1962. He was valedictorian of the College of Engineering. He attended Stanford University in Palo Alto, CA, graduating with an MS degree in electrical engineering in 1963. He then pursued a Ph.D. degree in electrical engineering at the University of Utah in Salt Lake City, graduating in 1967. He was awarded a Special Postdoctoral Fellowship from the National Institutes of Health to study bioengineering, which he took at the University of Washington in Seattle from 1972 to 1974. In addition, he has conducted research at the University of California at Santa Barbara and at Cornell University in Ithaca, NY.

Dr. Christensen was appointed an assistant professor of electrical engineering at the University of Utah in 1971, where also received an appointment as an assistant professor of bioengineering in 1974. He was chairman of the Bioengineering Department from 1985 to 1988. He currently is a professor in both departments.

His industrial experience includes Bell Telephone Laboratories in Murray Hill, NJ; IBM in San Jose, CA; Hewlett-Packard Co. in Palo Alto, CA; and General Motors Research Laboratories in Santa Barbara, CA. He has also been a consultant for several companies. His research interests range from electromagnetics to optics to ultrasound. He did early work on a fiber-optic temperature probe used for monitoring temperature during electromagnetic hyperthermia and has worked in numerical techniques for electromagnetic applications, mainly using the finite-difference time-domain method, including its use in optics. He wrote a textbook entitled *Ultrasound Bioinstrumentation* and has been co-director of the Center of Excellence for Raman Technology at the University of Utah, where he received the Outstanding Teaching Award and the Outstanding Patent Award from the College of Engineering. His recent interests have been in biomedical optics, especially for sensing and imaging applications.

Carl H. Durney was born in Blackfoot, ID April 22, 1931. He received a BS degree in electrical engineering from Utah State University in 1958, and MS and Ph.D. degrees in electrical engineering from the University of Utah in 1961 and 1964, respectively.

From 1958 to 1959, Dr. Durney was an associate research engineer with the Boeing Airplane Co. in Seattle, WA, where he investigated the use of delay lines in control systems. He has been with the University of Utah since 1963, where he is presently professor emeritus of electrical engineering and professor emeritus of bioengineering. From 1965 to 1966, he worked in the area of microwave avalanche diode oscillators at Bell Telephone Laboratories in Holmdel, NJ, while on leave from the University of Utah. He was visiting professor at the Massachusetts Institute of Technology doing research in NMR imaging and hyperthermia for cancer therapy during the 1983–84 academic year while on sabbatical leave from the University of Utah. At the University of Utah, until he retired in 1997, Dr. Durney taught and conducted research in electromagnetics, engineering pedagogy, electromagnetic biological effects, and medical applications of electromagnetics.

Dr. Durney is or has been a member of the Institute of Electrical and Electronics Engineers (IEEE), the Bioelectromagnetics Society, Commissions B and K of the International Union of Radio Science (URSI), Sigma Tau, Phi Kappa Phi, Sigma Pi Sigma, Eta Kappa Nu, and the American Society for Engineering Education (ASEE). He served as vice president (1980–81) and president (1981–82) of the Bioelectromagnetics Society, as a member (1979–88) and chairman (1983–84) of the IEEE Committee on Man and Radiation (COMAR), as a member of the American National

Standards Institute C95 Subcommittee IV on Radiation Levels and/or Tolerances with Respect to Personnel (1973–88), as a member of the editorial board of the IEEE Transactions on Microwave Theory and Techniques (1977–1997), and as a member of the editorial board of Magnetic Resonance Imaging (1983–1995). He was a member of the National Council on Radiation Protection and Measurements from 1990–1996. He served as a member of the Peer Review Board on Cellular Telephones (Harvard Center for Risk Analysis) from 1994–1997. In 1980, Dr. Durney received the Distinguished Research Award, and in 1993 the Distinguished Teaching Award from the University of Utah. In 1982, he received the ASEE Western Electric Fund Award for excellence in teaching and the Utah Section IEEE Technical Achievement Award. Utah State University named him College of Engineering Distinguished Alumnus in 1983. In 1990, the Utah Engineering Council named him Utah Engineering Educator of the Year. He was elected a fellow of the IEEE in 1992. In 1993, the Bioelectromagnetics Society awarded him the d'Arsonval Medal.

Dedication

---

to
Marie and Laraine

Contents

Chapter 5   Dosimetry

Chapter 6   Examples of Medical Applications of Electromagnetic Fields

1 Electric and Magnetic Fields: Basic Concepts

1.1 INTRODUCTION

All of classical electromagnetics stems from the phenomenon that electric charges exert forces on one another. The concepts of electric and magnetic fields are used to describe the multitude of complex effects that result from this basic phenomenon. Although classical electromagnetic (EM) field theory is typically couched in vector calculus and partial-differential equations, many of the basic concepts and characteristic behaviors can be understood without a strong mathematical background. This book describes and explains these basic concepts and characteristic behaviors with a minimum of mathematics. This chapter explains and discusses the basic concepts of electric and magnetic fields as a basis for what follows in the remainder of the book.

1.2 ELECTRIC-FIELD CONCEPTS

A fundamental law called Coulomb's law states that electric charges exert forces on one another in a direction along the line between the charges. Charges with the same sign repel, and charges with opposite signs attract. The magnitude of the force exerted on one charge by another charge is inversely proportional to the square of the distance between the two charges. Because keeping track of the forces exerted on individual charges in a complex system of charges is impossible in practice, the concept of electric field is used to account for the forces.

The concept of electric field is illustrated by this thought experiment: Place a point test charge Q_{test} at a point in space P, as shown in Figure 1.1(a). Other charges that exist will exert a force on the test charge. Measure that force. Let the force be denoted by **F**. By definition, the *electric field strength* at point P is given by

$$\mathbf{E} = \frac{\mathbf{F}}{Q_{test}} \tag{1.1}$$

as shown in Figure 1.1(b). (The direction of **E** is the direction of the force exerted on a positive test charge. The force on a negative test charge such as an electron would be in the opposite direction.) Thus **E** is a force per unit charge. **E** is also called *electric field intensity*, or often just electric field*. The units of **E** are volts/meter (V/m).

Because **F** is a vector, **E** is also a vector. A vector is a quantity that has both a direction and magnitude. In this book, vectors are denoted by boldfaced symbols. The direction of a vector is represented by an arrow, as in Figure 1.1. The magnitude of a vector is represented by the same symbol as the vector but not boldfaced. For example, let us define a vector **v** as a velocity having a direction from south to north and a magnitude of 30 meters/second. Then the magnitude of **v** is expressed as v = 30 meters/second. Similarly, E is the magnitude of the vector **E**.

---

* Throughout the book, the symbol **E** stands for either "electric," or "electric field." Similar notation is used for other vector fields. In each case, the meaning will be clear from the context.

0-8493-7686-6/97/$0.00+$.50
© 1997 by CRC Press LLC

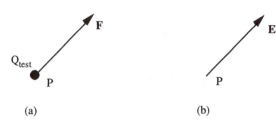

FIGURE 1.1 (a) Force **F** exerted on a charge Q_{test} placed at a point P in space. (b) Electric field **E** at the point P defined as $\mathbf{E} = \mathbf{F}/Q_{test}$.

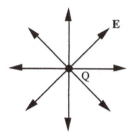

FIGURE 1.2 Plot of the electric field produced by a single point charge Q.

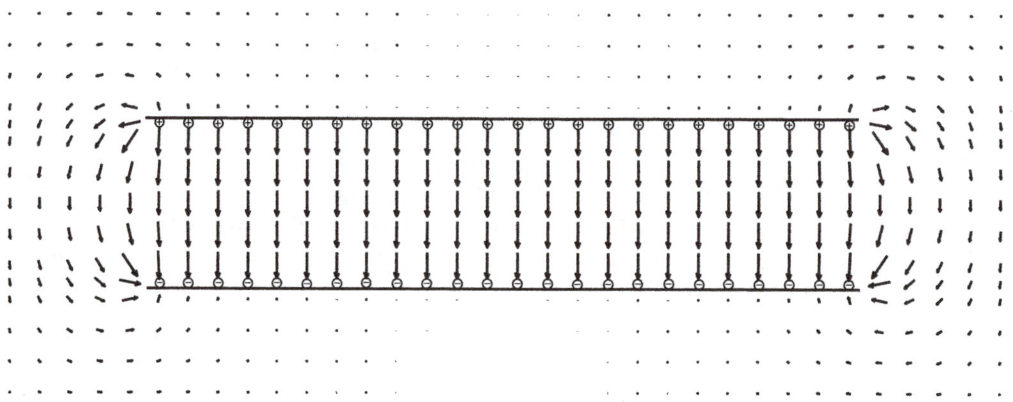

FIGURE 1.3 The **E** field produced by two uniform sheets of charge, positive charge on the top and negative charge on the bottom. This configuration is similar to a parallel-plate capacitor.

As a consequence of the definition of electric field, a charge q placed in an electric field **E** will experience a force given by $\mathbf{F} = q\mathbf{E}$. The larger the **E**, the larger the force **F** exerted on the charge q. The fundamental effect of an electric field on a body placed in it is to exert forces on the charges in that body, as explained in Section 1.6.

Electric fields are represented graphically in two ways. Figure 1.2 illustrates the first method, using the electric field produced by a single point charge Q as an example. Remember that **E** fields are produced by charges. The **E** produced by a single point charge is perhaps the simplest example of an **E** field. In this first method of displaying **E** fields, the direction of **E** is shown by arrows, and the magnitude of **E** is indicated by the closeness of the arrows. In areas where the arrows are close together, the magnitude is higher than in areas where the arrows are farther apart. For example, near the charge, the arrows are close together, indicating a large E. Farther away from the charge, the arrows are farther apart, indicating a smaller E.

The second method of representing vector fields such as **E** is illustrated in Figure 1.3, which shows the **E** field produced by two uniform sheets of charge. In this method, the direction of the

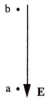

FIGURE 1.4 Configuration for calculating the potential difference of point b with respect to point a in the presence of **E**.

E field is also shown by arrows. The magnitude of **E** is indicated by the length of the arrows. The longer the arrow, the larger the E. This second method is often used when the **E** fields are calculated by numerical methods and plotted by computer graphical methods; this is the method used most often in this book. The **E** field produced by the two uniform sheets of charge is uniform near the center of the sheets. At the edges of the sheets, the **E** bends around, or "fringes."

Because **E** fields exert forces on charges, work is required to move charge from one point in space to another in the presence of an **E** field. The work done per unit charge is called *electric potential difference*. Electric potential difference is often referred to as potential difference, or just "voltage," because its unit is the volt (V). When **E** is known as a function of space, the potential difference between any two points can be calculated. Consider first the simplest case when **E** is uniform in the space between two points and a positive charge is moved from one point to another along a path in the opposite direction of **E**, such as moving a charge from point *a* to point *b* in Figure 1.4. For this case, the potential difference of point b with respect to point a is given by

$$V_{ba} = Ed \tag{1.2}$$

where d is the distance between the two points. Electrical potential difference refers to potential energy. If a charge were moved from point *a* to point *b*, it would possess potential energy, because if it were released, the force produced on it by **E** would cause it to move, thus converting its potential energy to kinetic energy. When the **E** field is not uniform or when the path between *a* and *b* is not in the opposite direction of **E**, Equation 1.2 does not apply and a more complicated calculation is required. Familiar devices such as 12-volt automobile batteries and 1.5-volt dry cells are used to produce potential differences. Large electric generators produce the potential differences that we use for a multitude of purposes in our homes.

When **E** does not vary with time or when it varies slowly with time (the frequency is low), the work done in moving charge between two points is independent of the path over which charge is moved between the two points. In this case, the **E** field is said to be a *conservative* field, and the potential difference is a unique quantity. When **E** varies rapidly with time (the frequency is high), the work done in moving charge between two points generally depends upon the path over which charge is moved between the two points, and a unique potential difference cannot be defined. In this case, **E** is not a conservative field. In special cases (see Section 3.5.1), **E** can vary rapidly with time and still be a conservative field.

Moving charges produce *electric current*, which is defined as the time rate of change of charge. The unit of charge is the coulomb (C). Current at a given point in space is the amount of charge passing that point per second. The unit of current is the ampere (A). Thus, one ampere equals one coulomb per second. *Current density* is defined as current per unit area. Its units are amperes/square meter (A/m^2).

If a time-constant potential difference V is applied between two points and a total current I flows between the two points as a result of the applied voltage, then the current is given by I = V/R, where R is the *resistance* (units are ohms) between the two points. As its name implies, resistance opposes the flow of current. This relationship is called *Ohm's law*; it is one of the fundamental laws of electric circuit theory.

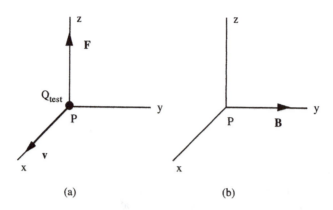

FIGURE 1.5 (a) Force **F** exerted on a test charge having velocity **v** at a point P in space. **F** is perpendicular to **v**. (b) Magnetic flux density **B** defined at point P to account for **F**.

The electric field shown in Figure 1.3 could also be produced by replacing the two sheets of charge with metal plates and applying a potential difference between the two by connecting, for example, a battery between the plates. The potential difference would produce current through the battery, transferring charge from one plate to the other and thus producing charged plates that would be equivalent to the configuration of Figure 1.3.

1.3   MAGNETIC-FIELD CONCEPTS

In the previous section, electric field concepts were explained as a means of accounting for the forces between charges that act on a line between the charges. When charges move, they exert another kind of force on one another that is not along a line between the charges. Magnetic fields are used to account for this other kind of force. The concept of magnetic flux density **B** is illustrated by the following thought experiment: Measure the force on a test charge having velocity **v** at a point P in space, as illustrated in Figure 1.5(a). The *magnetic flux density* **B** is defined as having a magnitude given by $B = F/vQ_{test}$ and a direction that is perpendicular to both **v** and **F**, as shown in Figure 1.5(b). The unit of **B** is the tesla (T). Magnetic flux density is often referred to as just "magnetic field."

As a consequence of the definition of **B**, a charge q having a velocity of **v** and placed in a field **B** will experience a force having a magnitude qvB and a direction that is perpendicular to both **v** and **B**.

Figure 1.6 shows vector plots of the **B** produced by a line current (an infinitely long current) and by a loop current. The **B** produced by the line current is strongest near the current, as indicated by closer spacing of the arrows. In each case, the **B** lines encircle the current, a characteristic that is described in more detail in Section 1.5.

1.4   SOURCES OF E FIELDS (MAXWELL'S EQUATIONS)

Because **E** fields are defined to account for the forces exerted by charges on one another, the fundamental sources of **E** fields are electric charges. Specific information about how charges act as sources for **E** fields is given by Maxwell's equations, which are a fundamental set of equations that form the framework of all of classical electromagnetic field theory. Although the mathematical content of this book is minimized, Maxwell's equations are stated below because they are so fundamental and so famous in electromagnetics that readers should be introduced to them, even if they might not have a background in vector calculus and partial-differential equations. The qualitative meaning of these equations will be explained without giving the mathematical details.

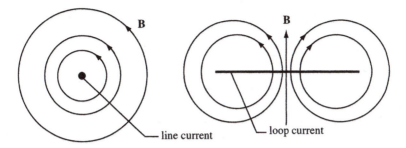

FIGURE 1.6 **B** fields produced by a line current and a loop current. The diagram shows just the edge of the loop current.

Two of Maxwell's equations describe sources of **E**: one source is a time-varying **B** field, and the other is charge density ρ. Each source produces **E** fields with specific characteristics. For clarity, we describe these when each source acts alone, but in general the **E** is produced by a combination of sources.

The first of Maxwell's equations that we discuss is

$$\nabla \times \mathbf{E} = -\partial \mathbf{B}/\partial t. \tag{1.3}$$

$\nabla \times \mathbf{E}$ is a mathematical expression called the curl of **E**. $\partial \mathbf{B}/\partial t$ is the time rate of change of **B**. Equation 1.3 means that a changing **B** field is a source of **E** and that the **E** field produced by the changing **B** encircles it. Therefore, a time-changing **B** acts as a source of electric field. Generally speaking, the greater the time rate of change of **B**, the stronger **E** field it produces.

Figure 1.7 shows an example of the **E** fields in a nonmetallic container of saline produced by a changing **B** as calculated from a 2D model. The **E**-field lines encircle the changing **B**, which is directed out of the paper. Figure 1.8 shows the same configuration with an object added to the saline that has a higher conductivity (see Section 1.6) than the saline. Here again the **E**-field lines tend to encircle the changing **B**, but they are modified by the presence of the small object that has higher conductivity. The higher conductivity of the small object causes the **E** fields inside the object to be weaker than those in the saline. The **E**-field pattern in the small object can be thought of as consisting of two components: (1) the globally circulating **E** field of Figure 1.7 without the small object, and (2) an **E**-field component circulating locally around the center of the small object. The resulting net pattern is a combination of the two, as shown in the magnified view of the object in Figure 1.9. On the left side and near the top of the object, the globally circulating **E** tends to cancel with the locally circulating **E**, while on the right side and near the bottom of the object, the two fields tend to add, producing a circulating pattern offset from the center of the object.

A second of Maxwell's equations, which describes the **E** produced by charge density, is

$$\nabla \bullet \mathbf{E} = \frac{\rho}{\varepsilon} \tag{1.4}$$

The expression $\nabla\bullet\mathbf{E}$ is called the divergence of **E**. ρ is electric charge density in coulombs/meter³ (C/m³), and ε is a parameter called *permittivity* (see Section 1.6). Equation 1.4 means that electric charge is a source of **E** and that the **E** lines begin and end on charges.

Figure 1.10 shows an example of the **E** fields produced by charges. A potential difference applied between a long wire and a metal plate produces positive charges on the wire and negative charges on the plate. These charges produce the kind of **E**-field lines shown.

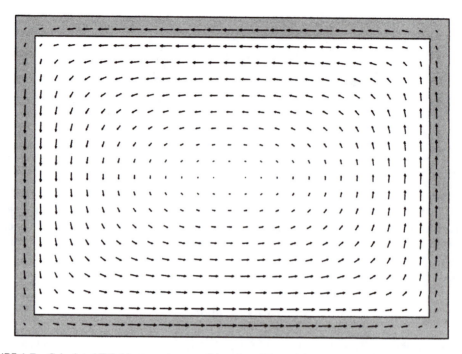

FIGURE 1.7   Calculated **E** fields at one instant of time for a 2D model consisting of a 1-kHz **B** field (directed out of the paper) applied to a nonmetallic container of saline.

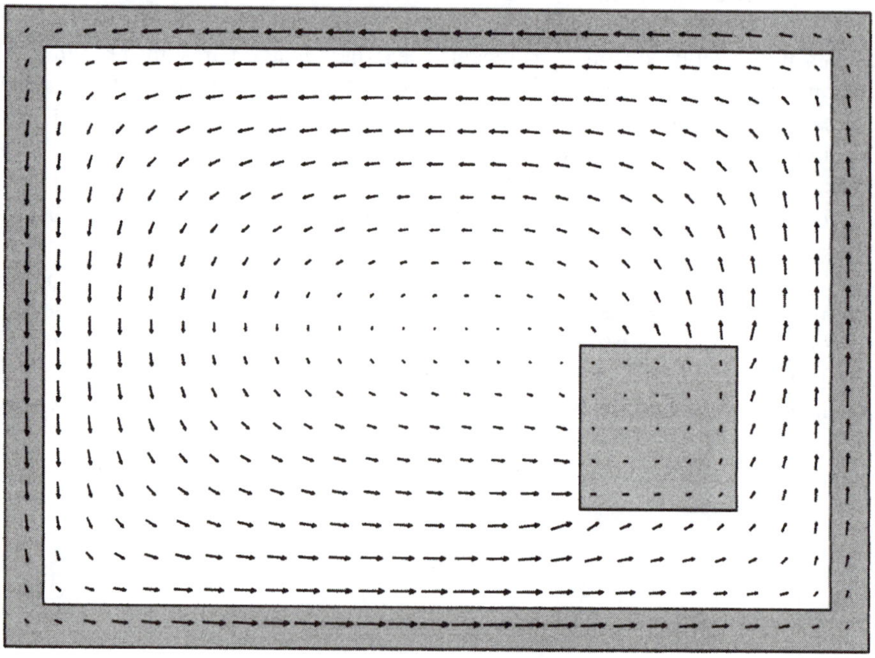

FIGURE 1.8   The same configuration as in Figure 1.7 but with an object of higher conductivity placed in the saline.

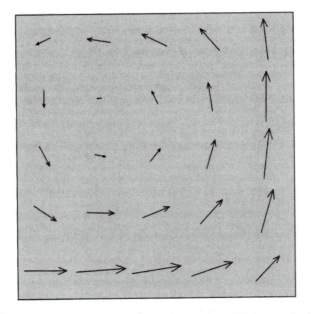

FIGURE 1.9   A magnified view of the E fields in the small object of higher conductivity of Figure 1.8.

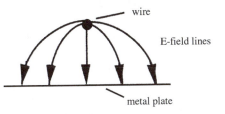

FIGURE 1.10   The E field produced by positive charges on a wire and negative charges on a metal plate resulting from a potential difference applied between them.

1.5   SOURCES OF B FIELDS (MAXWELL'S EQUATIONS)

Two other Maxwell's equations describe sources of **B**. The third equation states that

$$\nabla \times \mathbf{B} = \mu\left(\mathbf{J} + \varepsilon\frac{\partial \mathbf{E}}{\partial t}\right), \tag{1.5}$$

where μ is a constant called *permeability* (Section 1.6). This equation means that current density **J** and a time-changing electric field $\partial \mathbf{E}/\partial t$ are both sources of **B** and that the **B**-field lines produced by these two sources encircle **J** and $\partial \mathbf{E}/\partial t$. And finally, the last of Maxwell's equations is

$$\nabla \bullet \mathbf{B} = 0. \tag{1.6}$$

This equation states that the divergence of **B** is always zero, which means that there are no magnetic charges analogous to electric charges and that **B**-field lines always occur in closed loops, since they do not begin and end on charges, as do **E** fields.

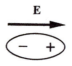

FIGURE 1.11   Illustration of how an **E** causes charge separation, which results in an electric dipole, the combination of a positive and a negative charge separated by a very small distance.

Figure 1.6 shows examples of how current density **J** produces **B** fields and how the **B**-field lines encircle the current. At low frequencies, the time-changing **E** field is usually a weak source compared with **J**, so typical low-frequency systems do not involve significant **B** fields produced by $\partial\mathbf{E}/\partial t$. Therefore, we postpone discussion of examples showing how $\partial\mathbf{E}/\partial t$ produces **B** until Chapter 3.

1.6   ELECTRIC- AND MAGNETIC-FIELD INTERACTIONS WITH MATERIALS

One of the more important aspects of electromagnetics is how electromagnetic fields interact with materials; for example, how **E** and **B** fields affect the human body. Because **E** and **B** were defined to account for forces among charges, the fundamental interaction of **E** and **B** with materials is that **E** and **B** exert forces on the charges in the materials. The interaction is even more complicated than that, though, because the charges in materials also act as sources of **E** and **B**. The "applied" fields, as they are often called, are produced by source charges external to a given material in the absence of the material. The "internal" fields are the combination of the applied fields and the fields produced by the charges inside material. The "scattered fields" are fields external to the object but produced by charges inside the object. Usually, in an electrically neutral object, the algebraic sum of the positive and negative charges inside the object is zero, and the positive and negative charges are microscopically so close together that the fields they produce cancel on a macroscopic scale. The applied fields, however, exert forces on the internal charges, which causes them to separate so that the macroscopic fields they produce no longer cancel. These fields combine with the original applied fields to produce a new internal field, which further affects the internal charges. This process continues until an equilibrium is reached, resulting in some net internal field.

In most cases, accounting for the interaction on a microscopic scale with charges in a material is impossible in practice. The interaction is therefore described macroscopically in terms of three effects of fields on the charges in material: induced polarization, alignment of already existing electric dipoles, and movement of "free" charges. Figure 1.11 illustrates the concept of induced dipoles. Before the **E** is applied, the positive and negative charges are so close together that the macroscopic fields they produce cancel each other. When an **E** field is applied, the positive charge moves in one direction and the negative in the opposite direction, resulting in a slight separation of charge. The combination of a positive and a negative charge separated by a very small distance is called an *electric dipole*. The creation of electric dipoles by this separation of charge is called *induced polarization*.

In some materials, electric dipoles already exist, even in the absence of an applied **E** field. These permanent dipoles are randomly oriented, so the net fields they produce are zero. When an **E** field is applied, the permanent dipoles partially align with the applied **E**, as illustrated in Figure 1.12. The applied **E** exerts a force on the positive charge of the dipole in one direction and on the negative charge in the opposite direction, causing the dipole to rotate slightly and thus partially align with the applied **E**. This partial alignment of the permanent dipoles reduces the randomization so that the net **E** field produced by the collection of dipoles is no longer zero.

The third effect of applied **E** fields on material charges is illustrated in Figure 1.13. Some charges (electron and ions) in materials are "free" in the sense that they are loosely bound and can move in response to an applied **E** field. These charges move a short distance, collide with other particles, then

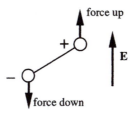

FIGURE 1.12 Illustration of partial alignment of a permanent electric dipole by an applied **E** field.

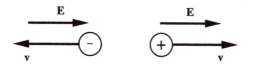

FIGURE 1.13 "Free" charges in materials acquire a velocity in response to an applied **E** field. Positive charges move in the same direction as **E**, and negative charges move in a direction opposite to the direction of **E**.

move in a different direction, resulting in some macroscopic average velocity in the direction of the applied **E** field. The movement of these charges constitutes a current that is called "*conduction current.*"

Similarly to how **E** causes partial alignment of permanent electric dipoles in materials, **B** causes partial alignment of permanent magnetic dipoles in materials, but there is no effect of **B** similar to separation of electric charge by an applied **E** field.

Because the interactions of **E** and **B** with materials are too complex to keep track of in terms of individual charges, three parameters are defined to account for these interactions on a macroscopic scale. Induced polarization and alignment of permanent electric dipoles is accounted for by *permittivity*, which describes how much induced polarization and partial alignment of permanent electric dipoles occurs for a given applied **E**. Conduction current is accounted for by *conductivity*, which describes how much conduction current density will be produced by a given applied **E**. Alignment of permanent magnetic dipoles is accounted for by *permeability*, which describes how much partial alignment of permanent magnetic dipoles occurs for a given applied **B**.

Permittivity is often represented by the Greek letter epsilon (ε); its units are farads/meter (F/m). The permittivity of free space (no charges present) is called ε_0 and in the International System of Units (SI), $\varepsilon_0 = 8.854 \times 10^{-12}$ F/m. *Relative permittivity* is defined as $\varepsilon_r = \varepsilon/\varepsilon_0$. It is the permittivity relative to that of free space, and it is unitless. Conductivity is often represented by the Greek letter sigma (σ); its units are siemens per meter (S/m). The relationship between current density **J** and electric field is $\mathbf{J} = \sigma\mathbf{E}$. Permeability is usually represented by the Greek letter mu (μ); its units are henrys/meter (H/m). The permeability of free space is $\mu_0 = 4\pi(10^{-7})$ H/m, and *relative permeability* is defined as $\mu_r = \mu/\mu_0$; it is unitless.

For sinusoidal steady-state fields (Section 1.10), a special method (see Section 1.11) of solving Maxwell's equations results in the definition of quantities called *complex permittivity* and *complex permeability*. A complex number is one containing the square root of (-1), which we designate as $j = \sqrt{-1}$ (see Section 1.11). Complex permittivity is defined as

$$\varepsilon = \varepsilon_0\left(\varepsilon' - j\varepsilon''\right)$$

where, as explained above, ε_0 is the permittivity of free space, and the quantity $(\varepsilon' - j\varepsilon'')$ is called the complex *relative permittivity*. The meaning of ε' and ε'' is discussed in the next section.

Complex permeability is defined as

$$\mu = \mu_0\left(\mu' - j\mu''\right)$$

where μ_0 is the permeability of free space, and the quantity $(\mu' - j\mu'')$ is called the *complex relative permeability*. The meaning of μ' and μ'' is also discussed in the next section.

1.7 ENERGY ABSORPTION

In many, but not all, electromagnetic field interactions, energy transfer is of prime consideration. The **E** field can transfer energy to electric charges through the forces it exerts on them, but the **B** field does not transmit energy to charges. The forces that **B** exerts on the charges can change their directions, but not their energy, because these **B**-field-exerted forces are always in a direction perpendicular to the velocities of the charges. The **B** field can, however, transfer energy through forces on permanent magnetic dipoles. Because biological tissue is mostly nonmagnetic (contains very few permanent magnetic dipoles), this latter effect is not prominent in EM biological interactions.

For the special case of sinusoidal steady-state EM fields, the time rate of energy transferred to charges in an infinitesimal volume element ΔV of a material is given by

$$P = \left(\sigma + \omega\varepsilon_0\varepsilon''\right)E^2_{\mathrm{rms}}\Delta V \text{ watts (W)} \tag{1.7}$$

where ω is the radian frequency in radians/second (r/s) (Section 1.10), and E_{rms} is the root-mean-square (rms) value (Section 1.12) of the magnitude of **E** *at that point*. Thus Equation 1.7 is a *point relation* because it applies only at the given point where **E** has that particular value. The time rate of energy change is called *power*, which has units of watts (W). The unit of energy is the joule (J). One watt is equal to one joule per second. Since ΔV has units of m³, the quantity $(\sigma + \omega\varepsilon_0\varepsilon'')\,E^2_{\mathrm{rms}}$ has units of W/m³, which is the density of absorbed power.

The *specific absorption rate* (SAR) is defined as the time rate of energy transferred divided by the mass of the object. "Specific" refers to the normalization to mass, and "absorption rate" refers to the rate of energy absorbed by the object. For the special case of the sinusoidal steady-state EM fields, the time-average SAR is given by

$$SAR = \left(\sigma + \omega\varepsilon_0\varepsilon''\right)\frac{E^2_{\mathrm{rms}}}{\rho} \text{ watts/kilogram (W/kg),} \tag{1.8}$$

where ρ is the mass density in kg/m³. Again, Equation 1.8 is a point relation, so it is often called the *local* SAR. The *space average* SAR for a body is obtained by calculating the local SAR at each point in the body and averaging over the whole body.

From Equation 1.8, we see that the SAR varies directly as both σ and ε'', or in other words, σ and ε'' indicate how much energy will be absorbed by the material for a given **E**. Because losses are often associated with power absorption, σ and ε'' are said to be indicators of the *lossiness* of materials. The greater the σ or the ε'', the greater the loss in the material; that is, the more power is absorbed for a given **E**. Generally speaking, tissue with higher water content, such as muscle, is more lossy than drier tissue, such as bone and fat.

Dielectrics are nonmetallic materials, i.e., materials with negligible conduction current (negligible σ). The properties of dielectrics are often described in terms of the *loss tangent*, or *dissipation factor*, which is defined as

$$\tan\delta = \frac{\varepsilon''}{\varepsilon'}. \tag{1.9}$$

Tables of dielectric properties often give ε' and $\tan\delta$.

Another common definition is that of *effective conductivity*, which is defined as

$$\sigma_{eff} = \left(\sigma + \omega\varepsilon_0\varepsilon''\right), \tag{1.10}$$

where σ_{eff} has units of siemens/meter (S/m). Thus in terms of effective conductivity, the SAR is given by

$$SAR = \frac{\sigma_{eff}E^2_{rms}}{\rho} \text{ W/kg.} \tag{1.11}$$

Materials are often characterized by ε' and σ_{eff}, where σ_{eff} is frequently referred to as just "conductivity." In terms of the peak value of **E** (see Equation 1.22 and the discussion in connection with Equation 1.17), the SAR is given by

$$SAR = \frac{\sigma_{eff}E^2}{2\rho} \text{ W/kg.} \tag{1.12}$$

1.8   OTHER ELECTROMAGNETIC FIELD DEFINITIONS

Two other definitions are used in electromagnetic field theory. One is *magnetic field strength* or *magnetic field intensity*, defined as

$$\mathbf{H} = \frac{\mathbf{B}}{\mu}, \tag{1.13}$$

which has units of ampere per meter (A/m). As discussed in Chapter 3, **H** is often more convenient to use than **B** in describing EM wave interactions. In practice, both **B** and **H** are often referred to simply as magnetic fields.

The other definition is *electric flux density* or *electric displacement*, defined as

$$\mathbf{D} = \varepsilon\mathbf{E}, \tag{1.14}$$

which has units of coulombs per square meter (C/m²). Sometimes using **D** is more convenient than **E** in EM field theory, but this book mostly uses **E**.

1.9   BOUNDARY CONDITIONS

Boundary conditions are relationships between EM fields that must be satisfied at the interface between two different materials, as required by Maxwell's equations. Because these boundary conditions are useful in interpreting and explaining characteristic behaviors of EM field interactions with biological systems, they are discussed here.

Figure 1.14 illustrates the boundary conditions on the **E** field. Because **E** is a vector, it can be resolved into two components: one parallel (tangential) to the boundary and one perpendicular (normal) to the boundary. Resolving vectors into components is explained in Figure 1.15, which illustrates how the vector **A** can be resolved into different pairs of components that are perpendicular (normal) to each other. Vectors are added graphically tail-to-head. Thus, the tail of $\mathbf{A}_2$ is placed at the head of $\mathbf{A}_1$ and then the sum of $\mathbf{A}_1$ and $\mathbf{A}_2$ is a vector from the tail of $\mathbf{A}_1$ to the head of $\mathbf{A}_2$, which in Figure 1.15(a) is the vector **A**. $\mathbf{A}_1$ and $\mathbf{A}_2$ are normal to each other. Figure 1.15(b) shows

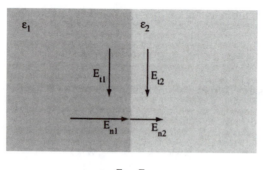

$$E_{t1} = E_{t2}$$
$$\varepsilon_1 E_{n1} = \varepsilon_2 E_{n2}$$

FIGURE 1.14 Illustration of conditions of the **E** field required by Maxwell's equations to be satisfied at the interface (boundary) between two media with different permittivities.

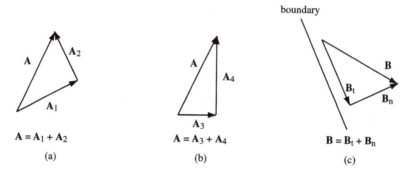

$$A = A_1 + A_2 \qquad\qquad A = A_3 + A_4 \qquad\qquad B = B_t + B_n$$

(a) (b) (c)

FIGURE 1.15 Resolving vectors into components. (a) **A** is resolved into components A_1 and A_2. (b) **A** is resolved into components A_3 and A_4. (c) **B** is resolved into components B_t and B_n.

how two other vectors, A_3 and A_4, add up to the same vector **A**. A_3 and A_4 are also normal to each other. Thus, **A** can be *resolved* into the components A_1 and A_2. **A** can also be resolved into components A_3 and A_4, as well as into many other components. Figure 1.15(c) shows how the vector **B** can be resolved into two components B_t and B_n, where B_t is the component that is tangential (parallel) to a given boundary line and B_n is the component that is normal to the boundary line.

Maxwell's equations require that the normal components of the **E** field at a charge-free boundary satisfy this equation:

$$\varepsilon_1 E_{n1} = \varepsilon_2 E_{n2}, \qquad\qquad (1.15)$$

where E_{n1} is the normal component of the **E** field in medium 1 *at the boundary*, and E_{n2} is the normal component of the **E** field in medium 2 *at the boundary*. Note that Equation 1.15 is required to be true only at the interface, or boundary, between the two media. The **E** field may change significantly as a function of position in the medium, and Equation 1.15 is not required to be satisfied at any points other than those on the boundary.

The boundary condition for the tangential components of **E** at the boundary is

$$E_{t1} = E_{t2}, \qquad\qquad (1.16)$$

where E_{t1} and E_{t2} are the tangential components of **E** *at the boundary* in medium 1 and medium 2, respectively.

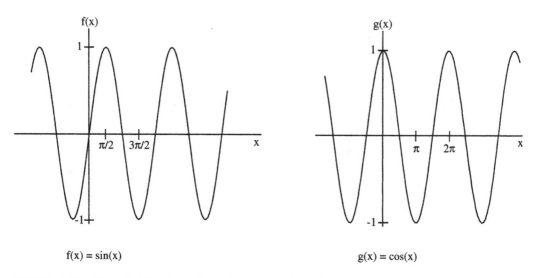

f(x) = sin(x)   g(x) = cos(x)

FIGURE 1.16 Sinusoidal functions of x, a sine wave and a cosine wave.

As an example of the boundary conditions, suppose that medium 1 in Figure 1.14 is air, and medium 2 is muscle tissue. At low frequencies, $\varepsilon_2/\varepsilon_1 \approx 10^6$. From Equation 1.15, this means that $E_{n2}/E_{n1} \approx 10^{-6}$. The normal **E** field in the muscle at the boundary would therefore be much smaller than the normal **E** field in the air at the boundary. On the other hand, from Equation 1.16, the tangential components of **E** in the air and in the muscle are equal at the boundary. Because the **E** in the air is a combination of incident and scattered fields (Section 1.6), it is difficult to draw conclusions about the relative magnitudes of the internal **E**-field components compared with the incident **E**-field components from boundary conditions alone. It turns out, though, that when the incident **E** is mostly normal to biological tissue at low frequencies, the internal **E** is smaller than when the incident **E** is mostly parallel to biological tissue, as will be explained in more detail later.

1.10 SINUSOIDAL EM FUNCTIONS

Sinusoids, or *sinusoidal wave functions*, are widely used to describe behaviors in physical systems, including electromagnetic systems. Figure 1.16 shows a sine wave, f(x) = sin(x), and a cosine wave, g(x) = cos(x). x is called the *independent variable* and f and g are *dependent variables*. These functions are both called sinusoids because they are described by the trigonometric functions sin(x) and cos(x). Values of the functions sin(x) and cos(x) for various values of x can be found in mathematical books and tables and from engineering and scientific calculators.

In electromagnetics, typical independent variables are space and time. We will use time as the independent variable in describing the properties of sinusoids. When time is the independent variable, the function is said to be in the *time domain*. Any sinusoidal function of time can be written in the general form

$$g(t) = G_m \cos(\omega t - \phi), \tag{1.17}$$

where G_m is called the *amplitude*, the *peak value*, or the *maximum value*, ω is the *radian frequency*, and ϕ is the *phase angle*. Figure 1.17 shows g(t) plotted both as a function of t and as a function of ωt. The *period* T is defined as the time between any two corresponding similar points on the waveform, such as between the two peaks in Figure 1.17(a). The frequency f is defined as

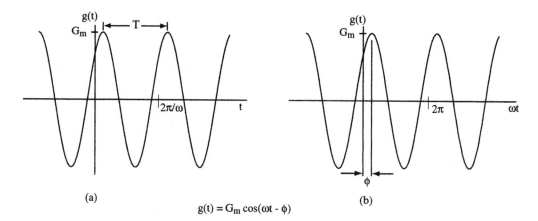

$$g(t) = G_m \cos(\omega t - \phi)$$

FIGURE 1.17 General form of a sinusoidal function or wave.

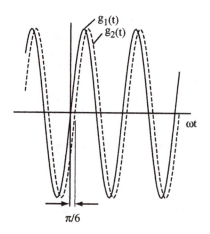

FIGURE 1.18 Two sinusoidal functions out of phase by $\pi/6$ radians.

$$f = \frac{1}{T} \qquad (1.18)$$

with units of hertz (Hz). The radian frequency (or angular frequency) ω is related to f by

$$\omega = 2\pi f \qquad (1.19)$$

with units of radians per second (r/s). You have probably noticed that $g(t) = G_m \cos(\omega t - \phi)$ is just $G_m \cos(\omega t)$ shifted to the right. Figure 1.17(b) shows that ϕ is the angle in radians by which $G_m \cos(\omega t)$ is shifted to the right to produce $G_m \cos(\omega t - \phi)$, when plotted against ωt. Note that when $\phi = \pi/2$ radians, $G_m \cos(\omega t - \pi/2)$ is exactly the same as $G_m \sin(\omega t)$. This illustrates the fact that any sinusoidal function of time can be written in the form of Equation 1.17.

Two sinusoids expressed in the form of Equation 1.17 are said to be *in phase* if their phase angles are equal. They are said to be *out of phase* when their phase angles are not equal. Figure 1.18 shows two functions, $g_1(t)$ and $g_2(t)$, that are out of phase by $\pi/6$ radians. Phase angles and differences in phase are often specified in degrees, just by converting the angles in radians to angles in degrees, although it is not strictly correct to do so because ωt has units of radians and ϕ and ωt must have the same units. (To convert from radians to degrees, multiply by $180/\pi$. To convert from degrees to radians, multiply by $\pi/180$.) Thus, $g_1(t)$ and $g_2(t)$ are said to be out of phase by $\pi/6$ radians or $30°$.

1.11   COMPLEX NUMBERS IN ELECTROMAGNETICS (THE PHASOR TRANSFORM)

When the sources in EM systems are sinusoidal functions, a powerful method called the *phasor transform* is usually used to solve the EM field equations. In this method, the electric and magnetic fields and other functions of interest are transformed from functions of time t to functions of radian frequency ω. They are said to be transformed from the *time domain* to the *frequency domain*, and the transformed functions in the frequency domain are called *phasors*. The phasor transform method consists of transforming all the EM functions and equations to the frequency domain, solving the transformed EM equations for the phasors, and then transforming the phasors back to the time domain to obtain the desired EM field quantities.

The method is advantageous because the EM equations in the frequency domain are algebraic equations. These are easier to solve than the corresponding equations in the time domain, which are partial-differential equations. One important consequence of the phasor transform is that the phasors are complex numbers. A complex number is a number that contains the square root of (−1), which we designate as $j = \sqrt{-1}$, and which is called an *imaginary number.*

A complex number consists of a real part and an imaginary part. For example, $3 + j2$ is a complex number: 3 is the real part, and j2 is the imaginary part. Electric-field phasors, for example, are often written as $E_r + jE_i$, where E_r is the real part and jE_i is the imaginary part.

The real and imaginary parts of phasors have important corresponding counterparts in the time domain. The time-domain function that corresponds to the real part of the phasor is 90° out of phase (see Section 1.10) with the time-domain function that corresponds to the imaginary part of the phasor. Thus j in the frequency domain is associated with a 90° phase shift in the time domain. The use of phasor transforms in EM field theory results in the definition of complex quantities such as complex permittivity and complex permeability (Section 1.6). Furthermore, boundary conditions similar to Equations 1.15 and 1.16 must be satisfied by the normal and tangential components of the phasor electric fields in the frequency domain. These are

$$\left(\sigma_1 + j\omega\varepsilon_1\right)\tilde{E}_{n1} = \left(\sigma_2 + j\omega\varepsilon_2\right)\tilde{E}_{n2} \tag{1.20}$$

$$\tilde{E}_{t1} = \tilde{E}_{t2} \tag{1.21}$$

at the boundary. In equations containing complex numbers, the real part of the left-hand side must be equal to the real part of the right-hand side, and the imaginary part on the left-hand side must be equal to the imaginary part on the right-hand side. The tilde above the E-field symbols indicates phasors in the frequency domain. These two relations show that both σ and ε have strong effects on the **E** fields.

The use of the phasor transform also results in the definition of *impedance*, which is the ratio of phasor voltage to phasor current. Impedance is like resistance in the sense that it opposes phasor current. That is, for a given phasor voltage, the phasor current is greater if the impedance is smaller. Impedance is different from resistance because it takes into account the effects of capacitance and inductance on phasor current. Impedance is defined only in the frequency domain; it is not defined in the time domain.

1.12   ROOT-MEAN SQUARE (RMS) OR EFFECTIVE VALUES

In many instances, it is convenient to describe time-varying fields in terms of their *root-mean-square* (rms) values. Of particular importance is the use of rms values in describing average power, as indicated in Equation 1.7. The basic reason for defining rms values is illustrated in Figure 1.19. The instantaneous power transferred to tissue by a time-varying **E** field is proportional to E^2 at any instant of time. For example, if **E** is a sinusoidal function of time, the instantaneous power

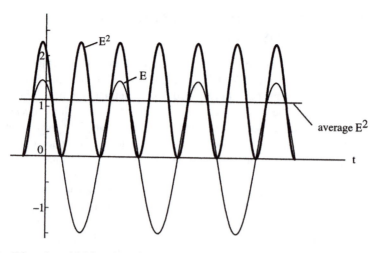

FIGURE 1.19   E is a sinusoidal function of t. Also shown is E^2. The average value of E^2 is one-half the peak value of E^2.

transferred will be proportional to the square of a sine wave, as shown in Figure 1.19. This instantaneous power fluctuates from zero to some maximum value that is proportional to the peak value of E^2. The average value of the power, which is usually of prime importance, is proportional to the average value of E^2, which is shown in Figure 1.19.

In the illustration in Figure 1.19, the peak value of E is 1.5, the peak value of E^2 is 2.25, and the average value of E^2 is 1/2 of 2.25, which is 1.125. The average value of E^2 can also be written as $(1.5/\sqrt{2})^2$. In this illustration, the quantity $(1.5/\sqrt{2})$ is the rms value of the function E. In general, the average value of the *square* of a sinusoidal function is equal to (peak value/$\sqrt{2}$)^2. Thus the rms value of any sine wave is its peak value divided by $\sqrt{2}$. For example, the rms value of **E** is

$$E_{rms} = \frac{E}{\sqrt{2}},$$ (1.22)

where E is the peak value of the **E** field. The rms value is also called the *effective value* because it has the same effect in producing average power as a steady function of the same value that does not vary with time.

In general, the rms value of a function is defined as the square root of the mean of the square of the function. Thus, to find the rms value of a given function, first square it, find the mean (average) of the squared function, then take the square root of that. For sinusoidal functions, this procedure always gives an rms value that is equal to the peak value divided by $\sqrt{2}$. As an example of finding the rms value of a nonsinusoidal function, calculate the rms value of the function f shown in Figure 1.20, which is a periodic function of x. First we square f as shown in the bottom of the graph. Then we find the average of f^2 by finding the area between f^2 and the x axis, which is shown shaded for one period of f in the figure. The area is $9 \times 1 + 4 \times 3 = 21$. The average value of f^2 is this area divided by the period (the period is 4). Thus, the average of f^2 is 21/4. The rms value of f is the square root of the average of f^2, which is $\sqrt{21}/2 = 2.29$.

1.13   WAVE PROPERTIES

For many physical configurations, the solutions to Maxwell's equations are most conveniently formulated in terms of propagating sinusoidal wave functions, or *waves*. Because an understanding

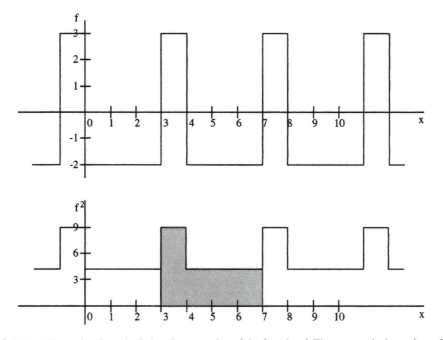

FIGURE 1.20 Illustration for calculating the rms value of the function f. The top graph shows f as a function of x, and the bottom one shows f^2 as a function of x.

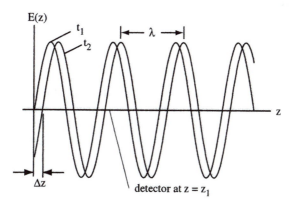

FIGURE 1.21 Illustration of a propagating wave. The magnitude of **E** is shown as a function of distance z at two different instants of time. The wave extends infinitely far in both the positive and negative z directions, though it is shown only over a limited range of z.

of the properties of waves is essential for much of the remainder of the book, those properties are reviewed here.

Figure 1.21 illustrates the concepts of propagating waves. As an example, the figure shows the magnitude of the electric field **E** as a function of distance z at two different instants of time, t_1 and t_2. These plots can be thought of as snapshots of a wave that is propagating to the right. The waveform shown is called a *sinusoidal wave* (see Section 1.10) because it is described by either the trigonometric function $\sin(\omega t - \beta z + \phi)$ or $\cos(\omega t - \beta z + \chi)$. ω is the *radian frequency* in radians per second (r/s), β is the *propagation constant* in inverse meters (m^{-1}), and ϕ and χ are called *phase angles*. The *wavelength* λ is defined as the distance in meters at one instant of time between any two corresponding points on the wave. In the figure, the two corresponding points are peaks (maxima) of the wave.

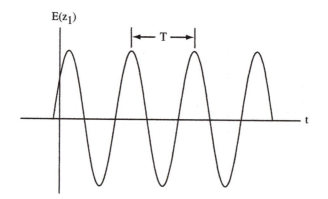

FIGURE 1.22   The output of a detector placed at position $z = z_1$ in Figure 1.21. The waveform extends infinitely far in both the positive and negative t directions, though it is shown only for a limited range of t.

The magnitude of the *phase velocity* v_p is defined as

$$v_p = \frac{\Delta z}{\Delta t},$$ (1.23)

where $\Delta t = t_2 - t_1$ is an infinitesimally small difference in time, and Δz is an infinitesimally small distance that the wave travels in the time Δt. The phase velocity, as its name implies, describes how fast the wave moves. The relationship between ω, β, and v_p is

$$\beta = \frac{\omega}{v_p}.$$ (1.24)

If a detector that registered the magnitude of **E** as a function of time were placed at a point z_1 on the z axis in Figure 1.21, the output of the detector as a function of time would be the sinusoidal function of time shown in Figure 1.22, with period T, frequency f, and radian frequency ω, as defined in Section 1.10. The wavelength, phase velocity, and frequency are related by

$$\lambda = \frac{v_p}{f}.$$ (1.25)

The phase velocity of a wave in free space is often designated by c. For planewaves (a specific kind of propagating wave that is described in Section 3.2.2) the phase velocity in free space is $c = 3 \times 10^8$ m/s. Combining Equations 1.19, 1.24, and 1.25 gives the relationship between the propagation constant β and the wavelength λ:

$$\beta = \frac{2\pi}{\lambda}.$$ (1.26)

Because sinusoidal functions are so prevalent in descriptions of electromagnetic fields, the characteristics of EM fields are often described in terms of the *frequency spectrum* or frequency range. Figure 1.23 shows a simplified representation of the electromagnetic frequency spectrum with both the frequency f and the wavelength λ in free space indicated. Some of the familiar frequency bands, such as the AM radio broadcast bands and the television broadcast bands are indicated in the figure. Maxwell's equations are valid over this whole range. It is astonishing,

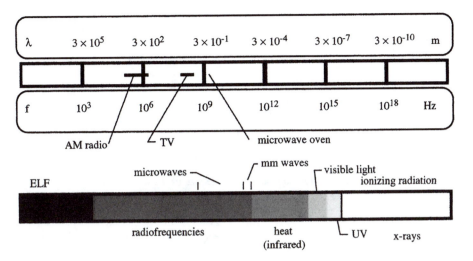

FIGURE 1.23   Simplified illustration of the extent of the electromagnetic frequency spectrum.

indeed, that one set of equations could be valid over more than 18 orders of magnitude in some parameter. Of course, even though Maxwell's equations apply over this whole range, and even though they are deceptively simple in form, they are certainly not easy to solve. No general solution that applies over the whole range is available. Instead, special techniques are used to find solutions for specific classes of problems in various frequency ranges. A general description of these techniques is given in the next section.

1.14   ELECTROMAGNETIC BEHAVIOR AS A FUNCTION OF SIZE AND WAVELENGTH

As explained in the previous section, Maxwell's equations apply over an extremely broad frequency spectrum. The characteristic behaviors of EM fields, however, are significantly different for different frequency ranges. To be more specific, the characteristic behaviors depend on the size of the EM device or system as compared to the wavelength. Suppose that L is the largest dimension of the device or system being considered and λ is the wavelength of the EM fields, then the techniques used to solve Maxwell's equations and the characteristic behavior of the EM fields can be summarized in terms of three categories, $\lambda \gg L$ (Figure 1.24), $\lambda \approx L$ (Figure 1.25), and $\lambda \ll L$ (Figure 1.26), as shown in Table 1.1. As a prelude to discussing the EM characteristic behaviors in each of these ranges, it needs to be pointed out that Equations 1.3 and 1.5 relate **E** and **B** in such a way that **E** and **B** are said to be *coupled*. That is, a time-changing **B** acts as a source of **E** (Equation 1.3), and in turn the time-changing **E** acts as a source of **B** (Equation 1.5). Thus when the fields vary with time, one cannot exist without the other, because each acts as a source of the other. When the fields do not vary with time, they are said to be *uncoupled*, because then they do not act as sources of each other.

When $\lambda \gg L$ (Figure 1.24), quasi-static EM field theory applies, which means that the spatial distribution of the EM fields over the extent of the device is the same as that of static fields, but the fields vary with time. **E** and **B** are said to be uncoupled when the $\partial \mathbf{E}/\partial t$ and $\partial \mathbf{B}/\partial t$ terms in Equations 1.3 and 1.5 are small enough to be neglected, which is often the case in this range. Therefore a **B** field can exist without a corresponding coupled **E** field. Also, an **E** field can be produced by charges, as described by Equation 1.4, without a corresponding coupled **B** field. In some configurations in this range, though, a time-varying **B** field can still produce a significant **E** field. In this case, the **E** field is, of course, produced by the **B** field. An example of this is shown in Figures 1.7–1.9.

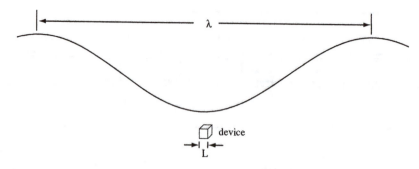

FIGURE 1.24   The wavelength is large compared with the size of the device.

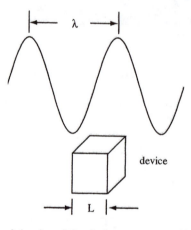

FIGURE 1.25   The wavelength and the size of the device are comparable.

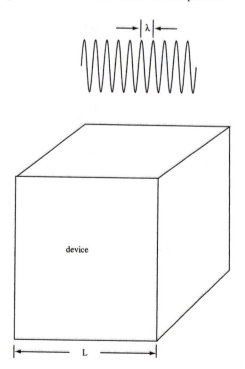

FIGURE 1.26   The size of the device is large compared with the wavelength.

TABLE 1.1
Summary of EM techniques and characteristics as a function of the relationship between device or system size L and wavelength λ.

When λ >> L (Figure 1.24)	Electric circuit theory and quasi-static EM field theory are used. Propagation effects are negligible. **E** and **B** are uncoupled. Energy is transmitted by wires and cables, but not in beams through the air.
When λ ≈ L (Figure 1.25)	Microwave theory is used. Propagation effects dominate. **E** and **H** are strongly coupled. Energy is transmitted through cables and hollow waveguides, and beamed through the air.
When λ << L (Figure 1.26)	Optics and ray theory are used. Propagation effects dominate. Energy is beamed through the air and is not transmitted through metallic cables or along metallic wires, but it can be transmitted through optical fibers.

In this range, a unique potential difference can be defined (see Section 1.2), and electric circuit theory (Kirchhoff's laws) is a good approximation to Maxwell's equations. Circuit theory is widely used in this range because it is much simpler than Maxwell's equations. Propagation effects are negligible in this range, and energy cannot be efficiently beamed through the air; it is transmitted along wires and through cables.

When λ ≈ L (Figure 1.25), that is, when the wavelength is of the same order of magnitude as the size of the system, EM field theory or microwave theory must be used. A unique potential difference cannot be defined in this range, except in special cases (see Section 3.5.1). Propagation effects dominate in this range, and **E** and **H** fields are described primarily in terms of propagating waves. **E** and **H** are strongly coupled. Neither **E** nor **H** fields can exist alone; the presence of one generates the other. Energy is typically transmitted along coaxial cables, through hollow pipes called waveguides, and beamed through the air. Calculations are often more difficult in this range than in the other two ranges because Maxwell's equations must be solved without powerful approximations like circuit theory or ray theory.

When λ << L (Figure 1.26), EM fields are described by optical theory, except at extremely high frequencies, where theories appropriate to x-rays are used. Ray theory is an approximation that is often used in optical theory. Again, propagation effects dominate here, and **E** and **H** are strongly coupled together. One cannot exist without the other. A unique potential difference can be defined in special cases, but the concept is rarely used in this range. Energy cannot be transmitted along wires in this range; it is typically beamed through the air or transmitted through dielectric waveguides such as optical fibers. This range includes the infrared, visible light, ultraviolet light, and x-ray portions of the EM spectrum. The upper frequency part of this frequency range is called the *ionizing radiation* range because the energy of the discrete energy-carrying packets of the EM wave, called photons, is great enough to cause ionization of atoms that the wave encounters, with corresponding danger to biological tissues.

Figure 1.27 shows again the EM spectrum with the addition of the characteristic ranges given in Table 1.1 for typical systems. The ranges are only approximate representations, and the transition from one range to another is gradual, not abrupt. Also, for some microcircuits, circuit theory may apply at higher frequencies than indicated in Figure 1.27 because L is very small for these circuits.

Figure 1.28 illustrates how the behavior of a common device, the screen in a microwave oven door, can be explained in terms of the characterizations of Table 1.1. When an EM signal is incident on a metal plate containing an array of holes of diameter d, the signal is mostly blocked when d << λ; the signal interacts strongly and passes through when d ≈ λ; and the signal passes through the holes almost freely when d >> λ. The screen in a microwave oven door typically contains holes with diameters on the order of 2 mm. The wavelength of the microwave EM fields generated by the oven is typically about 122 mm (frequency is 2450 MHz). The wavelength of the light produced by the light bulb in the oven is on the order of 0.5 micrometers (μm). The screen thus blocks the

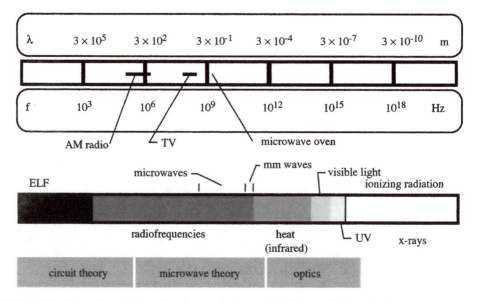

FIGURE 1.27 Illustration of how the characterizations of Table 1.1 fit into the frequency spectrum of Figure 1.23 for typical systems.

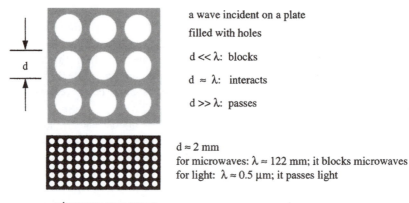

FIGURE 1.28 The behavior of the screen in a microwave oven door can be explained in terms of the characterizations of Table 1.1.

microwave signal because for it d << λ. On the other hand, the light passes through the holes almost freely because for it d >> λ. The screen, therefore, nicely contains the microwave energy but lets the visible light pass through so that the contents of the oven can be observed.

Because the characteristics of EM fields are so strikingly different in each of the three ranges described above, valuable insight can be gained by categorizing EM-field interactions in terms of these ranges. Accordingly, we describe EM-field behavior in each of these ranges in separate chapters, beginning in Chapter 2.

1.15 ELECTROMAGNETIC DOSIMETRY

Electromagnetic dosimetry consists of two main parts. First the incident **E** and **B** fields must be determined. Typically these fields are determined either from the nature of the sources producing them or by measurements. Second the **E** and **B** fields inside the object (typically humans or other

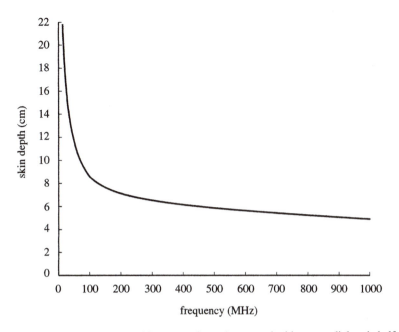

FIGURE 1.29   Skin depth as a function of frequency for a planewave incident on a dielectric halfspace having a permittivity and conductivity equal to two-thirds that of muscle tissue.

animals) must be determined, either by calculation or by measurement. The relationship between the incident EM fields and the internal EM fields is a strong function of the frequency of the incident fields, the size and shape of the body, and the electromagnetic properties of the body. Typically, different techniques are used to calculate and measure internal fields in each of the ranges described in Table 1.1. These techniques and typical results are described in subsequent chapters. In all cases, the relationship between the incident fields and the internal fields is very complicated.

In general, the penetration of incident fields into biological bodies decreases as frequency increases. This effect is illustrated by the graph in Figure 1.29, which shows the skin depth (defined below) as a function of frequency for a planewave incident on a dielectric halfspace having a permittivity and conductivity equal to two-thirds that of muscle tissue. Dielectric halfspace means half of all space is filled with one dielectric, and the other half is filled with another dielectric (often free space), with a planar interface between the two. Two-thirds the permittivity and conductivity of muscle were used because that is approximately the average of all the tissues in a typical human being. The skin depth is defined as the depth at which the EM fields have decreased to $1/e$ (0.37) of their value at the surface of the body (see Section 3.4.1), where $e = 2.718$ is the base of the natural logarithm. While the graph is for a dielectric halfspace, a similar effect occurs in humans and other animals. As the frequency is increased, the penetration generally becomes less and less. At optical frequencies, the penetration is very slight, and whatever effects the EM fields have on the body are primarily surface effects. Even at microwave frequencies, the penetration is relatively shallow.

2 EM Behavior When the Wavelength is Large Compared with the Object Size

2.1 INTRODUCTION

Chapter 1 explained that the characteristics of EM fields and their interactions with objects vary dramatically with the ratio of the wavelength of the EM fields to the object size. This chapter describes in detail the behavior of EM fields and their interaction with objects when the wavelength is large compared with the size of the object. As indicated by Figure 1.23, the wavelength in free space is 300 meters when the frequency is 1 MHz. Consequently, for objects about the size of people, the wavelength will be large in comparison with the object size at frequencies below 1 MHz. (Note that from Equation 1.25, the wavelength varies inversely as the frequency.) Thus the discussion in this chapter pertains mostly to the low-frequency region of the spectrum, including the commonly used power-line frequencies of 50 and 60 Hz, and what is referred to as the ELF band. The ELF (extra-low frequency) band is designated as the band of frequencies from 30 to 300 Hz.

2.2 LOW-FREQUENCY APPROXIMATIONS

Several useful approximations can be made when the wavelength is large compared with the size of the object. These approximations are often called low-frequency approximations because, as explained above, the frequency is typically low when the wavelength is large compared with the object size.

An important low-frequency approximation is electric-circuit theory, which is an approximation to Maxwell's equations (Sections 1.4 and 1.5). Voltage and current are the principal variables in electric-circuit theory, which consists of Kirchhoff's voltage and current laws, along with some auxiliary relations. Fortunately, electric-circuit theory is *much* simpler than EM field theory. It typically involves two scalar (nonvector) functions, voltage and current, that vary with time. EM field theory, on the other hand, typically involves electric and magnetic fields, both of which are vector functions that vary with three space variables as well as with time. Life would be difficult indeed if one had to solve Maxwell's equations for every situation in which circuit theory is commonly used.

The other main low-frequency approximation is called *quasi-static EM field theory*. In this approximation, the spatial variation of the **E** and **B** low-frequency fields is approximated as being the same as that of static (not varying with time) EM fields. This is a valuable approximation because the EM field equations are simpler for static fields than they are for time-varying fields. Quasi-static EM field theory is used whenever information about the **E** fields or **B** fields is needed. For example, it is used to calculate **E**-field patterns produced by high-voltage power lines operating at low frequencies. On the other hand, electric-circuit theory is used when the systems involve lumped elements such as resistors, capacitors, inductors, and transistors, in which case the distribution of the **E** and **B** fields is usually not needed.

An example of a quasi-static **E** field is one that is produced by a sinusoidally time-varying low-frequency potential difference applied between two parallel metallic plates. This potential difference produces an **E** field between the plates that is similar to that shown in Figure 1.3, but the pattern

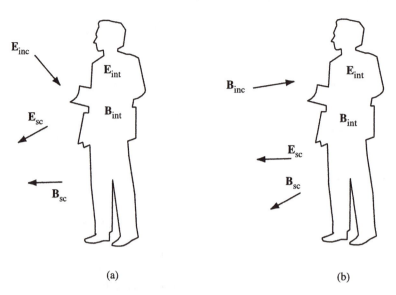

(a)   (b)

FIGURE 2.1   The internal and scattered **E** and **B** fields due to (a) the incident **E** alone and (b) the incident **B** alone.

as a whole varies sinusoidally with time. That is, the magnitude of the vector shown at each point changes sinusoidally with time in synchrony with all the other vectors, but the relative spatial pattern remains the same. This sinusoidal variation includes negative values (refer to Section 1.10 and Figure 1.16), which means that the vectors reverse directions periodically. In the example of the parallel-plate configuration, the **E** fields are found from the quasi-static approximation by solving the static EM field equations and then letting the resulting **E** vary sinusoidally with time. This is much easier than directly solving the time-varying EM field equations.

An important consequence of quasi-static field theory is that the **E** and **B** fields can exist independently, or they are said to be *uncoupled*. This can be seen from Maxwell's equations. As indicated by Equations 1.3 and 1.4, **E** can be produced by either a time-changing **B**, by a distribution of charges, or by both. It is important to note that a time-changing **B** is not necessary to produce the **E**, just charges. In fact, in the static case, $\partial \mathbf{B}/\partial t$ is zero and will not contribute to the **E**. In the quasi-static case, $\partial \mathbf{B}/\partial t$ is often (though not always) small enough to be neglected in comparison to contributions to **E** due to the charges. Thus a quasi-static **E** field can be produced by a charge distribution independently of any **B**, as indicated more specifically by Equation 1.4. Similarly, from Equations 1.5 and 1.6, when the $\partial \mathbf{E}/\partial t$ can be neglected in Equation 1.5, a **B** can be produced by a current independently of any **E**. On the other hand, in the high-frequency case, when the $\partial \mathbf{B}/\partial t$ and $\partial \mathbf{E}/\partial t$ cannot be neglected, Equations 1.3 and 1.5 show that **E** and **B** are coupled together, and one cannot exist without the other.

As a consequence of the quasi-static approximation, when the wavelength is large compared with the object size, the interaction of EM fields with objects can be described in terms of the two cases described in Figure 2.1. A typical situation consists of a set of sources that produces known EM fields in which an object is then placed. Some definitions are helpful: The *incident* **E** and **B** are the **E** and **B** fields produced by the sources without the object present. The *internal* **E** and **B** are the fields that exist inside the object. They consist of the original incident fields modified by the presence of the object. The *external* fields are the fields outside the object. They consist of the original incident **E** and **B**, plus the *scattered* **E** and **B**, which are the fields produced by the presence of the object in the incident fields. Sometimes the internal fields are of primary interest, and sometimes the scattered fields are of primary interest. At low frequencies, the internal fields are usually of most interest.

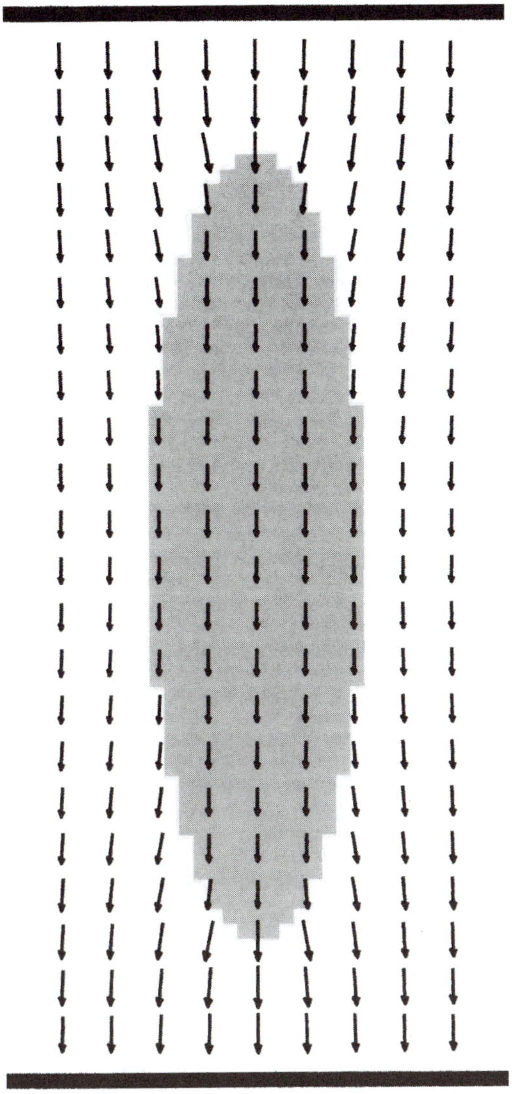

FIGURE 2.2 Calculated **E** fields in a 2D model of a prolate spheroid between two metallic plates, approximating a spheroid placed in a uniform **E** field. The **E** fields were calculated on a finer grid and displayed on a coarser grid to show more clearly the overall field pattern.

Because the **E** and **B** are uncoupled at low frequencies, the internal fields can be found by finding the internal **E** and **B** due to the incident **E** alone, and then finding the internal **E** and **B** due to the incident **B** alone, as illustrated in Figure 2.1. The total internal **E** is the vector sum of the internal **E** in (a) and the internal **E** in (b). A similar procedure can be used to find the internal **B** and the scattered **E** and **B**. Typical examples of each kind of internal field are given in the next sections.

2.3   FIELDS INDUCED IN OBJECTS BY INCIDENT E FIELDS IN FREE SPACE

Figure 2.2 shows the calculated internal **E** in a section of a simple two-dimensional model of a dielectric prolate spheroid placed in the uniform **E** (similar to that shown in Figure 1.3) that existed

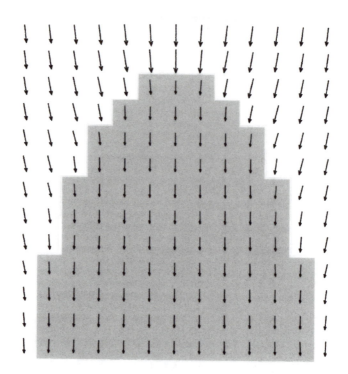

FIGURE 2.3 The field pattern around the top portion of the spheroid in Figure 2.2 as calculated on the finer grid.

between two metallic plates before the object was inserted. (A prolate spheroid has the shape of an egg.) When the spacing between the plates is large compared to the length of the body, this configuration produces approximately the same field pattern that occurs when the body is placed in a uniform **E** field in free space. In this numerical calculation (a finite-difference, frequency-domain solution of Maxwell's equations), the spacing between the plates was not made larger because that requires more computer memory, but the characteristics of the field patterns are approximately the same as those for a prolate spheroid placed in a uniform **E** in free space.

In Figure 2.2, the relative permittivity (see Section 1.6) of the prolate spheroid is $\varepsilon_r = 2$, which is a comparatively small value, since the relative permittivity of free space is 1. This comparatively small value of relative permittivity was used for illustrative purposes because larger values make the internal fields too small to be seen. The presence of the dielectric object perturbs the originally uniform **E** field in a way that can be thought of as the dielectric "pulling in" the **E**-field vectors. In smooth prolate spheroids, the **E** field inside is uniform in space. But in this model, in which the outer boundary is stair-stepped (a consequence of the numerical-calculation method), **E** is only approximately uniform because of the stair-stepping. The **E** vectors in Figure 2.2 were calculated on a finer grid but displayed on a coarser grid to show more clearly the overall field pattern. Figure 2.3 shows an enlarged view of the field pattern around the top portion of the spheroid as calculated on the finer grid. Note that the **E** field is weaker inside the object than outside.

The fact that **E** is weaker inside the dielectric than in the surrounding air can be explained in terms of the boundary conditions. As explained in connection with Equation 1.15 and Figure 1.14, the boundary conditions on **E** require that the normal component of **E** must be discontinuous at the boundary between two dielectrics by the ratio of the permittivities. In this case, if ε_1 is the permittivity of air and ε_2 is the permittivity of the spheroid, then Equation 1.15 requires that $E_{n2} = (\varepsilon_1/\varepsilon_2)E_{n1} = (1/2)E_{n1}$ *at the boundary*. From Figure 2.3, you can see that at the top of the

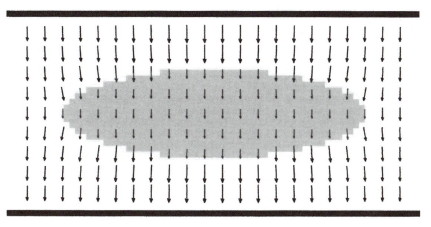

FIGURE 2.4   Calculated **E** fields in a model similar to that used in Figure 2.2 but with the long axis of the spheroid perpendicular to the originally uniform **E** in which it was placed.

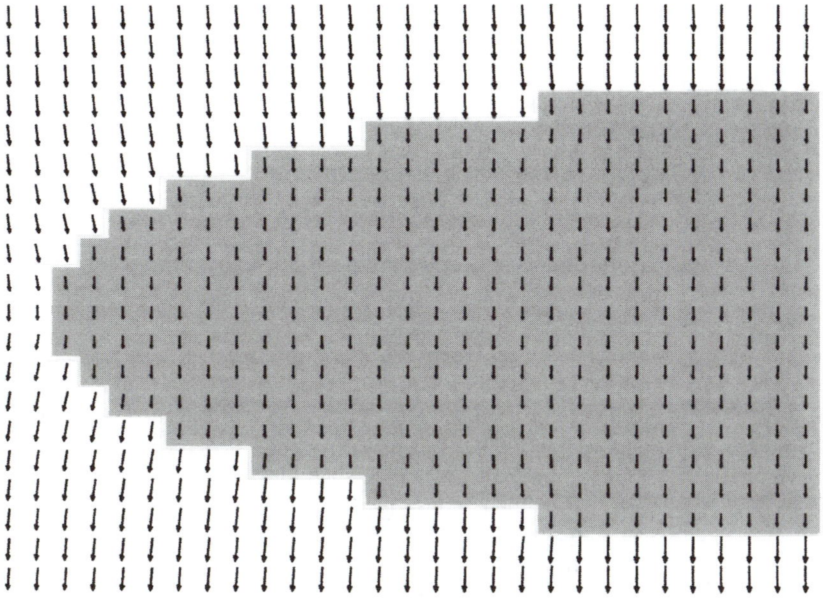

FIGURE 2.5   The field pattern near the left half of the spheroid in Figure 2.4 as calculated on the finer grid.

spheroid, the **E** fields are approximately normal to the boundary and that the normal component in the dielectric is about half that of the normal component in air. These fields are not the fields right at the boundary, but they are close enough to the boundary that they satisfy approximately the relationship required by the boundary conditions.

Figures 2.4 and 2.5 show the **E**-field patterns for a prolate spheroid with its long axis perpendicular to the originally uniform **E** field in which it is placed, essentially turned 90° with respect to the orientation of Figure 2.2. The behavior is similar, with the **E** fields weaker in the dielectric than in the surrounding air above and below the object.

If the permittivity of the dielectric were increased to a much larger value, the boundary conditions would require the normal **E** in the dielectric at the boundary to be much smaller than the normal **E** in the air at the boundary. This illustrates the following important characteristic of **E** fields in this low-frequency region of the spectrum: The **E** fields inside dielectric objects with

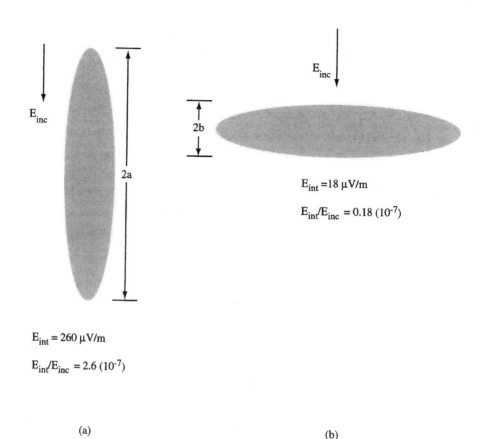

$$E_{int} = 260 \ \mu V/m$$

$$E_{int}/E_{inc} = 2.6 \ (10^{-7})$$

(a)   (b)

FIGURE 2.6 Comparison of the internal fields in two spheroids, (a) with the incident **E** parallel to the long axis of the spheroid, and (b) with the incident **E** perpendicular to the long axis of the spheroid. In both cases, the incident **E** is 1 kV/m, the conductivity is 0.067 S/m, the frequency is 60 Hz, a = 0.875 m, and b = 0.138 m. The internal **E** fields were calculated in 3D using a long-wavelength approximation to Maxwell's equations.

relatively high permittivities are usually much smaller than the **E** fields in the surrounding air. This behavior will be illustrated and explained further in subsequent sections.

Three-dimensional quasi-static solutions of Maxwell's equations in spheroidal coordinates for a prolate spheroidal model give more specific results about the internal fields in spheroidal objects, as illustrated in Figure 2.6, in this case for objects with more realistic relative permittivities near those of tissues. In both cases shown, the internal fields are six or seven orders of magnitude smaller than the incident field in which the objects were placed. This is attributable to the high permittivity and conductivity of the objects, which are approximate averages of all the tissues in the human body. Although the relative permittivity is of the order of 10^6, at this low frequency the conductivity probably dominates in determining the internal fields.

The ratio of the internal to incident **E** field for the case shown in (a) is almost 15 times greater than for the case shown in (b) even though the objects are the same in each case. This difference can be explained in terms of the boundary conditions. The incident field in (b) is "mostly normal" to the dielectric-air interface over a much larger portion of the surface of the body than it is in (a). Because the boundary condition as stated in Equation 1.15 requires the internal normal field to be smaller than the external normal field by the ratio of the permittivities, the internal field is smaller in (b) because the boundary condition forces it to be that way over a larger portion of the surface at the boundary.

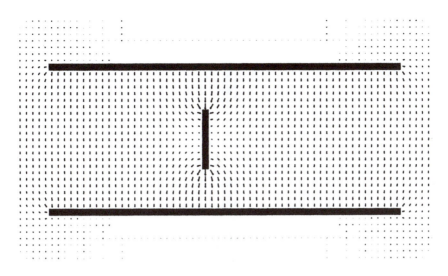

FIGURE 2.7 Calculated 2D E-field pattern for a slender metallic object placed in the originally uniform **E** between the capacitor plates.

2.4 E-FIELD PATTERNS FOR ELECTRODE CONFIGURATIONS

The previous section discussed the **E**-field effects of objects placed in uniform **E** fields in free space, as approximated by objects placed between metallic plates where the field was uniform before the object was placed there. This section discusses **E**-field effects produced by electrode configurations, such as those used in *in vitro* experiments.

2.4.1 CAPACITOR-PLATE ELECTRODES

An important characteristic of **E**-field interactions is illustrated in Figure 2.7, which shows the **E**-field pattern produced by a current source (not shown) connected between two metallic plates (a capacitor) in the presence of a slender metallic object. The presence of the object perturbs the otherwise uniform **E** field significantly, particularly near the sharp corners at its end. Figure 2.8 shows an enlarged view of the area around the object. This is an example of a general characteristic, that sharp corners and objects cause a concentration and enhancement of **E** fields, as required by the boundary conditions. This can be explained as follows: The high conductivity of the metal makes the **E** fields inside the metal very small. Since the tangential components of **E** must be equal at the boundary, the tangential **E** in the air at the boundary must therefore be very small, approximately zero. That means the **E** field in the air at the metal boundary must everywhere be normal to the metal. For the **E** to be normal to the metal everywhere around the corners, the **E**-field vectors must be crowded in, thus making the magnitude of **E** large. The more slender and pointed the object, the more the resulting concentration of **E** fields.

A similar effect is produced by dielectric objects, as illustrated in Figure 2.9, which shows a close-up view of the same capacitor arrangement as in Figure 2.7 but with a slender dielectric object having a relative permittivity of 100 instead of a metallic object. The dielectric has the effect of pulling the **E**-field lines into it (as in the spheroidal example in Section 2.3), thus distorting the otherwise relatively uniform fields and concentrating the **E** fields around the corners. An interesting example of this general effect would be you standing on the ground in a thunderstorm. The highly charged clouds produce a strong **E** field between the clouds and the earth, similar to the **E** produced between the metallic plates in Figure 2.7. You would be like the object between the plates,

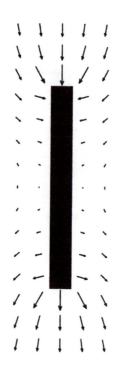

FIGURE 2.8 Expanded view of the region around the slender metallic object in Figure 2.7.

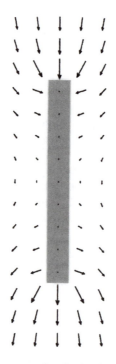

FIGURE 2.9 Expanded view of the region around a slender dielectric object with a relative permittivity of 100 placed between the capacitor plates in Figure 2.7.

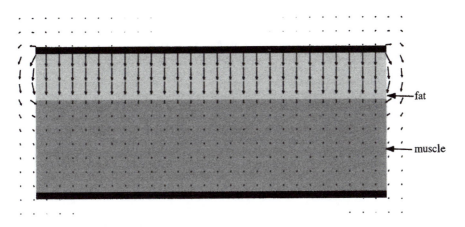

FIGURE 2.10 Calculated 2D E-field pattern at one instant of time for two layers of material having the electrical properties of fat and muscle placed between capacitor plates at 100 kHz.

concentrating the **E** field at the ends of your body. If you pointed a finger to the sky, the resulting more slender and pointed object would increase the concentration of the **E** field, perhaps enough to cause ionization and breakdown of the air, or, in other words, lightning. (Lightning rods are sharply pointed for this reason.) The best strategy in a thunderstorm is to make yourself as round and blunt as possible. Lying prone on the ground is not a good thing to do because you could be injured or killed by currents in the ground produced by the charged clouds.

Another interesting effect occurs when layers of different materials are placed between capacitor plates. Figure 2.10 shows the **E** fields that occur in two layers, one with a permittivity and conductivity similar to those of muscle and the other similar to those of fat. The **E** field in the fat is obviously much larger than the **E** field in the muscle. That should not be surprising, because the **E** fields in the two media are almost uniform and normal to the interface between the two materials. The boundary conditions (Equation 1.20) require that

$$\left(\sigma_f + j\omega\varepsilon_f\right)\tilde{E}_{nf} = \left(\sigma_m + j\omega\varepsilon_m\right)\tilde{E}_{nm} \tag{2.1}$$

at the boundary, where the subscript f refers to the fat and the subscript m to the muscle.

For these calculations, $\omega = 2\pi 10^5$ radians/second, $\sigma_f = 0.026$ S/m, $\varepsilon_f = 180\varepsilon_0$, $\sigma_m = 0.477$ S/m, and $\varepsilon_m = 5{,}758\varepsilon_0$. Since the conductivity and permittivity of muscle are both much larger than those of fat, the boundary condition requires that $\tilde{E}_{nm}$ be much smaller than $\tilde{E}_{nf}$. As a consequence, the fat is heated much more than the muscle, as described by Equation 1.11. Although σ_f is smaller than σ_m, the E_{rms} in the fat is greater than in the muscle, and since the SAR varies as E_{rms}^2, the SAR in the fat is considerably greater than in the muscle.

This simple example illustrates an important characteristic behavior: **E** fields normal to the interface between a high-permittivity material and a low-permittivity material produce high **E** fields in the low-permittivity material. This characteristic behavior explains why some EM applicators used to heat tumors for cancer therapy cause the fat to overheat; they produce **E** fields normal to the fat–muscle interface.

2.4.2 DISPLACEMENT CURRENT

The capacitor of Figure 2.11 illustrates another important concept: that of *displacement current*. The $\mathbf{J} + \varepsilon\partial\mathbf{E}/\partial t$ terms in Equation 1.5 represent total current density. Equation 1.5 is called a *point relation* because it describes the relationship between the fields at each point in the system. The **J** term is current density due to the movement of charges (conduction current density, see

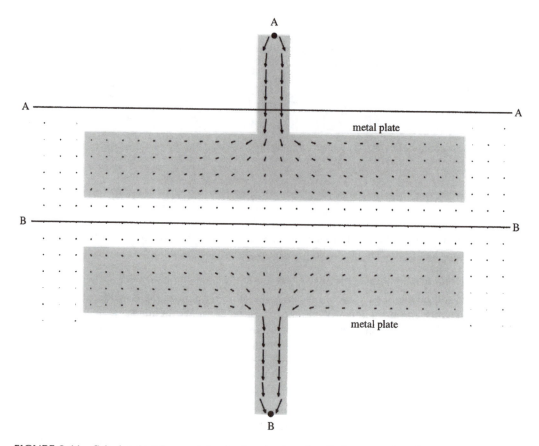

FIGURE 2.11   Calculated total current density (conduction plus displacement) in a 2D model of a parallel-plate capacitor with thick conductors (shown in gray) and empty space surrounding the conductors. A sinusoidal current source is connected between points A and B. The current density is shown at an instant of time when the current source is maximum.

FIGURE 2.12   A close-up view of the current density in the top conductor of the capacitor in Figure 2.11 (plotted to a different scale). Here, the current is predominantly conduction current.

Section 1.6), both at points in free space and at points in materials. The $\varepsilon\partial\mathbf{E}/\partial t$ term at points in free space does not involve movement of charge at all (since there are no free charges in free space), but it does have the same units as $\mathbf{J}$ (A/m²) and has the characteristics of a current density. It is called *displacement current density*. Including this term was the triumph of James Clerk Maxwell in formulating the famous equations named after him (Sections 1.4 and 1.5). At points in materials, $\varepsilon\partial\mathbf{E}/\partial t$ includes the effects of polarization (Section 1.6), but not those of "free" charge, which are included in the conduction current.

Figure 2.11 shows a vector plot of the total current density $\mathbf{J} + \varepsilon\partial\mathbf{E}/\partial t$ at an instant of time when the sinusoidal current source is a maximum. The conduction current density spreads out in the thick conducting plates, as shown in more detail in Figure 2.12. Figure 2.13 shows only the

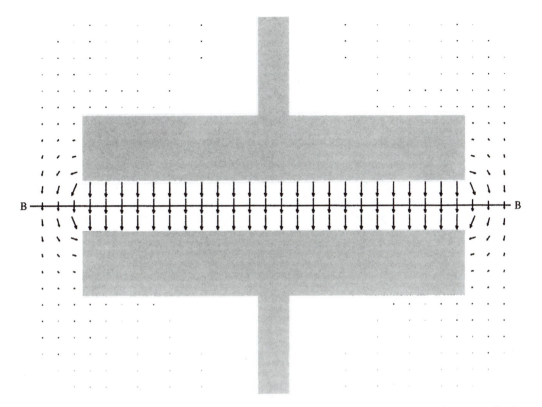

FIGURE 2.13 Calculated current density in the capacitor of Figure 2.11 but showing only the current density in the empty space surrounding the conductors plotted to a different scale from that of Figure 2.11. Here, the current is composed of displacement current only.

current density in the air between the plates and in the surrounding area, plotted to a different scale. The total current (current density times cross-sectional area) passing through *any* plane parallel to A-A in Figure 2.11 is the same and is equal to the current supplied by the current source. In plane A-A, the current consists of mostly the conduction current in the wire; the displacement current in the air is negligible. The total current passing through plane B-B in Figure 2.13, however, consists only of displacement current, for there are no charges present. This example shows how displacement current effectively continues current through space where no charges are present, making the total current (conduction plus displacement) continuous.

2.4.3 IN-VITRO ELECTRODE CONFIGURATIONS

An experimental configuration that is sometimes used in the laboratory to expose solutions to **E** fields is illustrated in Figure 2.14, which shows the **E** fields produced by two wire electrodes placed in a saline solution in a container with nonconducting walls. The figure shows the calculated **E** field in a 2D model. These results are similar to those of a 3D model looking down on the container from the top with the fields shown in a plane perpendicular to the electrodes. Figure 2.15 shows the fields just in the saline to give a closer view of the field pattern. The **E** fields are normal to the electrode surfaces and are somewhat uniform in the central region between the electrodes, but they are quite nonuniform in the regions around the electrodes. Figure 2.16 shows a close-up view of the region around the upper left corner of Figure 2.14. **E** fields are produced both in the container walls and in the space outside the walls.

A side view of the electrode configuration of Figure 2.14 is shown in Figure 2.17, which shows the calculated **E** fields in another 2D model. These 2D results are similar to those that would be

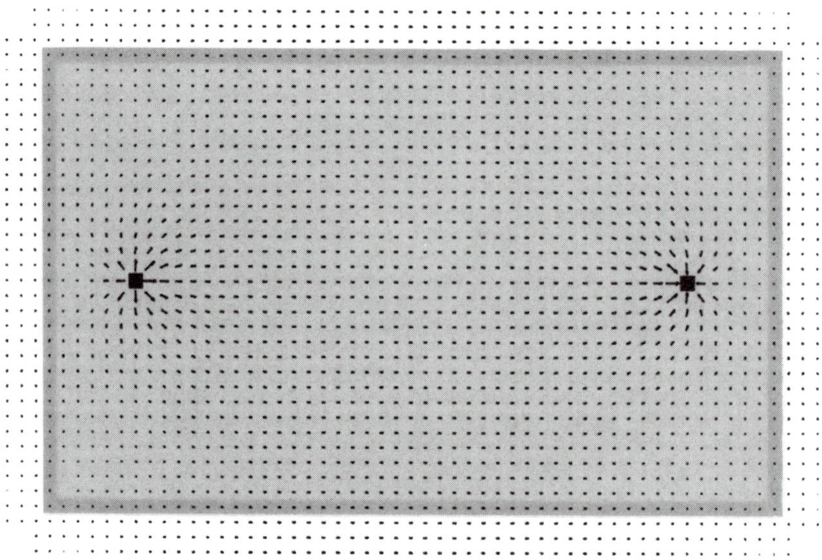

FIGURE 2.14 Calculated **E** fields in a 2D model of two wire electrodes (the black squares) placed in a saline solution in a nonconducting container. A 60-Hz sinusoidal current source is connected between the two electrodes. The **E** fields are shown at an instant of time when the current solution is a maximum.

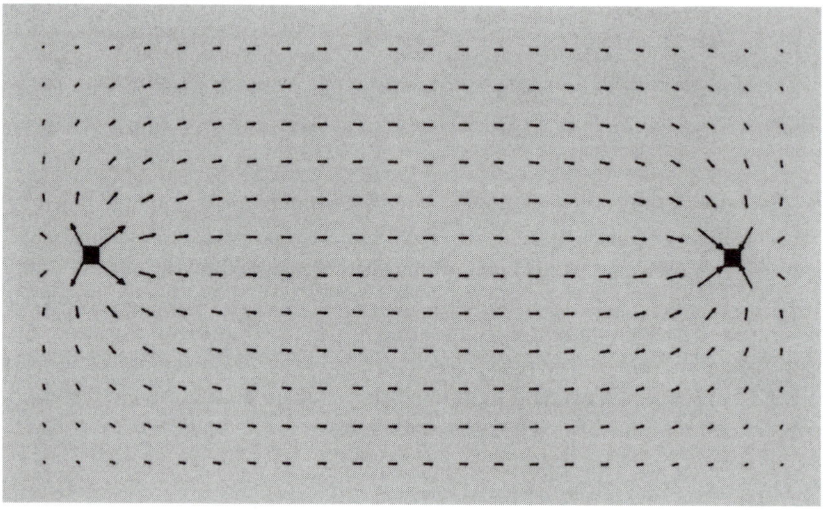

FIGURE 2.15 A close-up view of the **E** fields in just the saline of Figure 2.14 The **E** fields are interpolated and plotted on a coarser grid than in Figure 2.14 to show the field pattern more clearly.

obtained from a 3D model in a plane passing through the electrode centers. Figure 2.18 shows a close-up view of the fields just in the saline. The field pattern in this plane is quite uniform in between the electrodes, but again it is variable near the ends of the electrodes.

Figure 2.19 shows the effect of a nonconducting "bump" in the bottom of the nonconducting container. The nonconducting bump forces the current to flow around the bump in the saline, thus distorting the **E**-field pattern in its vicinity, as shown more clearly in the close-up view of Figure 2.20. The **E** field inside the bump is higher than in the surrounding saline for the same reason the fields in the fat of Figure 2.10 are higher than those in the muscle.

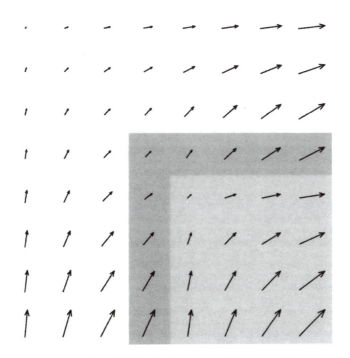

FIGURE 2.16 A close-up view of the **E** fields in the region of the upper left corner of Figure 2.14.

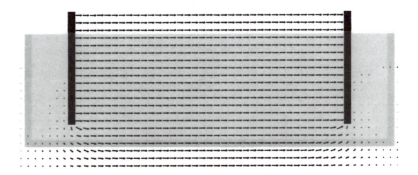

FIGURE 2.17 Calculated **E** fields in a 2D model of two wire electrodes (shown in black) placed in a nonmetallic container of saline (a side view). A 60-Hz sinusoidal current source (not shown) is connected between the two electrodes. The **E** fields are shown at an instant of time when the current source is a maximum.

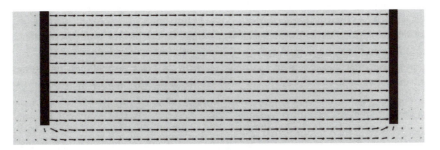

FIGURE 2.18 A close-up view of the **E** fields just in the saline of Figure 2.17.

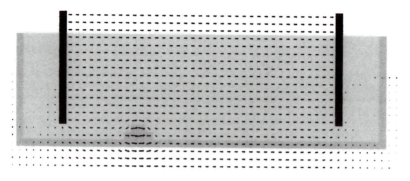

FIGURE 2.19   Calculated **E** fields in the model of Figure 2.17 but with a nonconducting "bump" on the bottom of the nonconducting container.

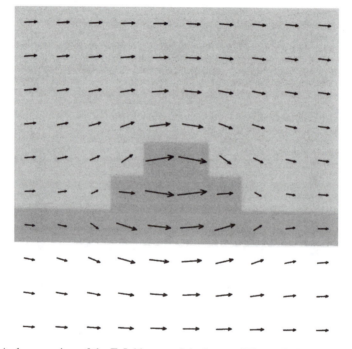

FIGURE 2.20   A close-up view of the **E** fields around the bump of Figure 2.19.

Another electrode configuration is shown in Figure 2.21, where the left electrode of Figure 2.14 has been replaced by a plate electrode. A closer view of the fields around the electrodes (Figure 2.22) shows how the **E** field is normal to the plate in the region just to the right of the plate, but is not much different from the pattern in Figure 2.14 around the wire electrode.

Two plate electrodes are shown in Figure 2.23, with a closer view shown in Figure 2.24. The **E**-field pattern between the plates is much more uniform than in any of the other configurations shown previously. This would be expected from the geometry of the configurations because the **E** fields must be normal to the metallic electrodes. Plate electrodes would obviously be a better choice in any experiment in which a uniform **E** field is desired.

Figures 2.25 and 2.26 show what happens when a coarse model of a nonconducting membrane enclosing a saline interior is placed between the plate electrodes of Figure 2.23. The nonconducting membrane forces current to flow around it, and the **E** fields in the membrane are much higher than in the surrounding saline for the same reasons as explained in connection with Figure 2.10. The fields in the saline region enclosed by the membrane are essentially zero, as seen in Figure 2.26.

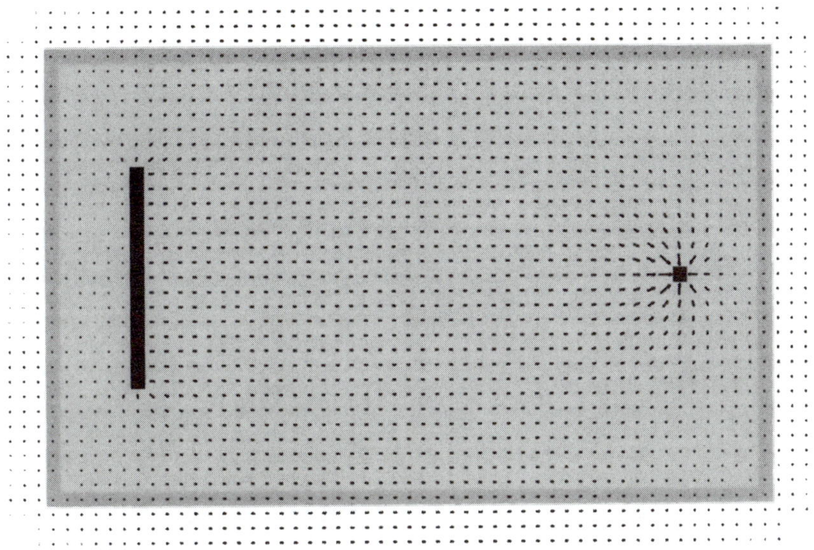

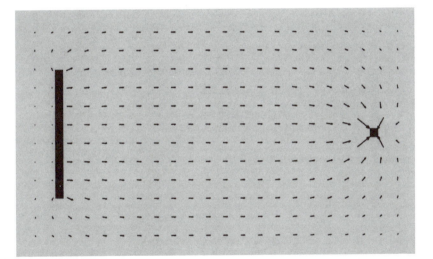

FIGURE 2.21 Calculated **E** fields in the model of Figure 2.14 but with the left wire electrode replaced by a plate electrode.

FIGURE 2.22 A close-up view of the **E** fields in the region near the electrodes of Figure 2.21. The **E** fields are interpolated and plotted on a coarser grid than in Figure 2.21 to show the field pattern more clearly.

The field patterns in Figures 2.14 through 2.26 illustrate the nature of the E-field patterns produced by various electrode configurations in solution. In some places, the **E** fields are approximately uniform over a limited region, but near the electrodes they are not close to being uniform, especially near small or pointed electrodes. These effects must be carefully taken into account when doing experiments in which the dosimetry of the **E** fields is important.

2.5 FIELDS INDUCED IN OBJECTS BY INCIDENT B FIELDS IN FREE SPACE

Figure 2.27 shows the calculated internal **E** in a simple 2D model of a conducting prolate spheroid placed in a 60-Hz sinusoidally time-varying and spatially uniform **B** field in free space. The **B** field

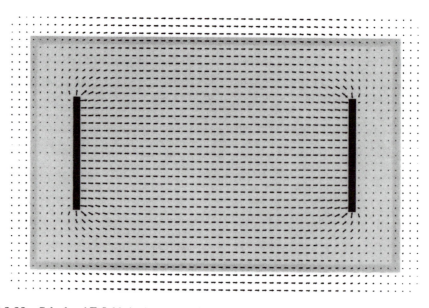

FIGURE 2.23 Calculated **E** fields in the model of Figure 2.21 but with the right wire electrode replaced by a plate electrode.

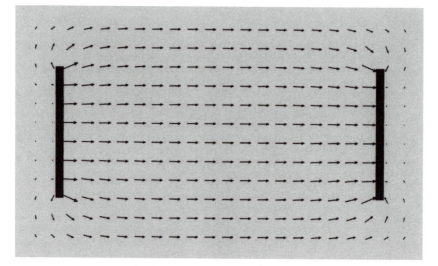

FIGURE 2.24 A close-up view of the **E** fields just in the saline of Figure 2.23. The **E** fields are interpolated and plotted on a coarser grid than in Figure 2.23 to show the field pattern more clearly.

in this case is directed out of the paper (the **B** field is parallel to the minor (short) axis of the spheroid, which is also directed out of the paper). As explained in Section 1.4, the time-varying **B** field produces **E** fields that encircle the **B** field. A close-up view of the **E** fields in the spheroid is shown in Figure 2.28. When the **B** field is parallel to the major (long) axis of the spheroid, the induced **E** field pattern is as shown in Figure 2.29, which shows one cross section of the spheroid, with the **B** field directed out of the paper. A view with a finer grid is shown in Figure 2.30. The pattern is similar in each cross section of the spheroid perpendicular to the major axis. As in the other orientation of the **B** field, the induced **E** field encircles the **B** field. Although the rectangular mathematical cells of the model do not represent the smooth boundaries of a prolate spheroid very well, the pattern of induced **E** fields is approximately the same as that for an actual prolate spheroid.

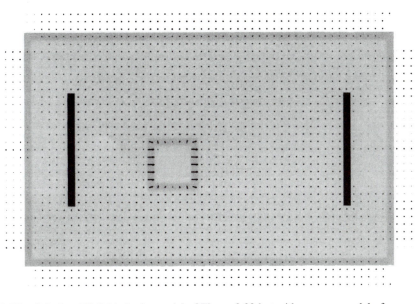

FIGURE 2.25   Calculated **E** fields in the model of Figure 2.23 but with a coarse model of a nonconducting membrane enclosing a saline interior placed in the saline between the plate electrodes.

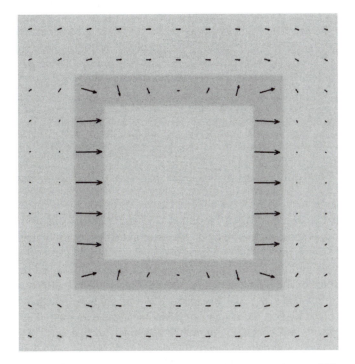

FIGURE 2.26   A close-up view of the **E** fields around and inside the membrane of Figure 2.25.

Figure 2.31 shows the results of 3D analytical calculations for the **E** fields induced in a prolate spheroid by a sinusoidally time-varying, spatially uniform **B** field. When the **B** field is parallel to the major axis of the spheroid, as shown in Figure 2.31(a), the induced E field in any cross section perpendicular to the major axis is given by $\omega Br/2$, where r is the distance from the spheroid major axis to the point at which the E field is evaluated, and ω is the radian frequency of the **B** field. The maximum E field induced by a B field of 1 mT at a frequency of 60 Hz is 25.8 mV/m, located at

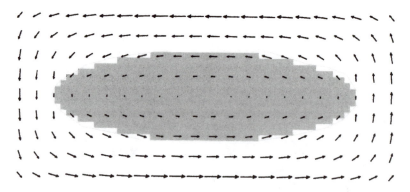

FIGURE 2.27 Calculated **E** fields in a cross section of a 2D model of a prolate spheroid in free space exposed to a uniform 60-Hz **B** field perpendicular to the major axis of the spheroid (i.e., **B** is directed out of the paper). The fields were calculated on a finer grid and displayed on a coarser grid to show the overall field pattern more clearly.

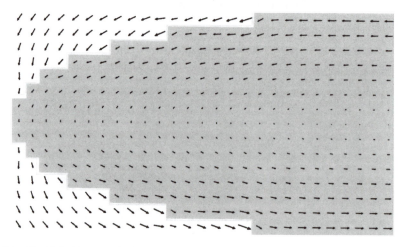

FIGURE 2.28 The E-field pattern in the left half of the spheroid in Figure 2.27 shown as calculated on the finer grid.

the outer surface of the spheroid. When the **B** field is parallel to the minor axis of the spheroid (Figure 2.31(b)), the maximum induced E field, located at the outer surface of the spheroid, is almost twice that value. The difference can be explained in terms of the cross-sectional area intercepted by the **B** field in each case. In Figure 2.31(a), the cross-sectional area intercepted by **B** is considerably less than that intercepted by the **B** field in Figure 2.31(b). This is an illustration of a general behavior: The **E** fields induced in a body by a spatially uniform **B** field are generally greater when the cross-sectional area intercepted by **B** is greater and are found near the outer periphery of the body.

The **E** fields induced in a coarse 2D model of an animal in free space exposed to a 60-Hz, spatially uniform **B** field are shown in Figure 2.32. Again, the **E** fields tend to circle around the applied **B** field, which is directed out of the paper. They are generally larger in the air surrounding the conducting tissue of the model than they are in the tissue. The **E** fields also tend to be small near the center of the system and larger around the outside, as in the spheroidal models. Figure 2.33 shows the **E** fields inside the model only (plotted to a different scale), where the circulating pattern is more obvious.

It is interesting to note that the **E** fields tend to circulate around the center of the trunk, but also to a lesser extent around the center of the head and the center of the legs. The circulation around the center of the left leg is shown more clearly in Figure 2.34, which shows just the left

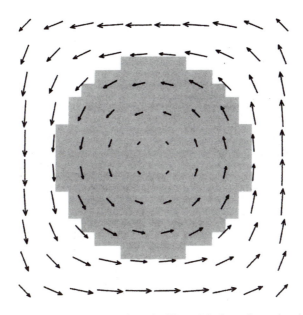

FIGURE 2.29   Calculated **E** fields in a cross section of a 2D model of a prolate spheroid in free space exposed to a uniform 60-Hz **B** field perpendicular to the minor axis of the spheroid (i.e., **B** is directed out of the paper). The fields were calculated on a finer grid and displayed on a coarser grid to show the overall field pattern more clearly.

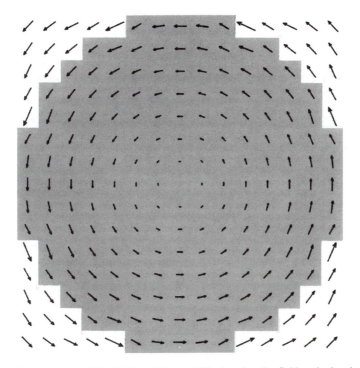

FIGURE 2.30   A close-up view of the fields in Figure 2.29, showing the fields calculated on the finer grid.

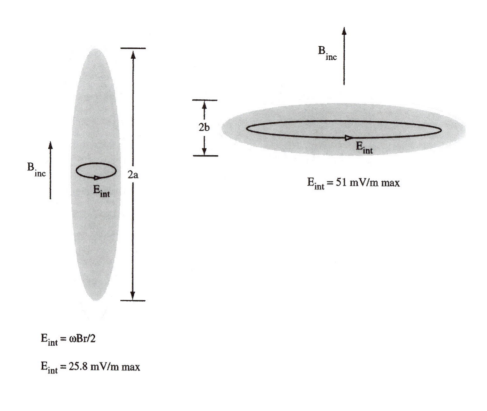

$$E_{int} = \omega Br/2$$

$$E_{int} = 25.8 \text{ mV/m max}$$

(a)   (b)

FIGURE 2.31 Comparison of the internal fields in two spheroids: (a) with the incident **B** parallel to the long axis of the spheroid and (b) with the incident **B** perpendicular to the long axis of the spheroid. In both cases, the incident **B** is 1 mT, the conductivity is 0.067 S/m, the frequency is 60 Hz, a = 0.875 m and b = 0.138 m. The internal **E** fields were calculated in 3D using a long-wavelength approximation to Maxwell's equations.

leg of Figure 2.33 still attached to the whole animal. Figure 2.35 shows the **E** fields in a leg that has been detached from the animal but exposed to the same **B** field and plotted to the same scale as in Figure 2.34. Although the fields at the very top of the detached leg are different from those of the attached leg, the fields at the bottom of the detached leg differ from those in the attached leg by less than one-half of 1%. This comparison indicates that the fields tend to circulate around the center of the attached leg as though it were a separate entity, and the fields are significantly different from those of a detached leg only in the region where the leg is attached. This effect becomes more pronounced as the leg becomes longer and thinner, and it becomes less pronounced as the leg becomes shorter and fatter (and blends more into the body as a whole).

Figure 2.36 shows a close-up view of just the **E** fields in the attached head and neck of the model of Figure 2.33. The pattern very clearly shows how the fields circulate around the center of the head almost as if it were detached. Only the fields near the neck are significantly different from those of a detached head. This effect becomes more pronounced as the area of the appendage becomes a greater portion of the entire area.

2.6 E-FIELD PATTERNS FOR *IN VITRO* APPLIED B FIELDS

In typical laboratory experiments, a biological sample is exposed to a **B** field produced by currents in a coil or a combination of coils, with the **B** field being approximately spatially uniform over the

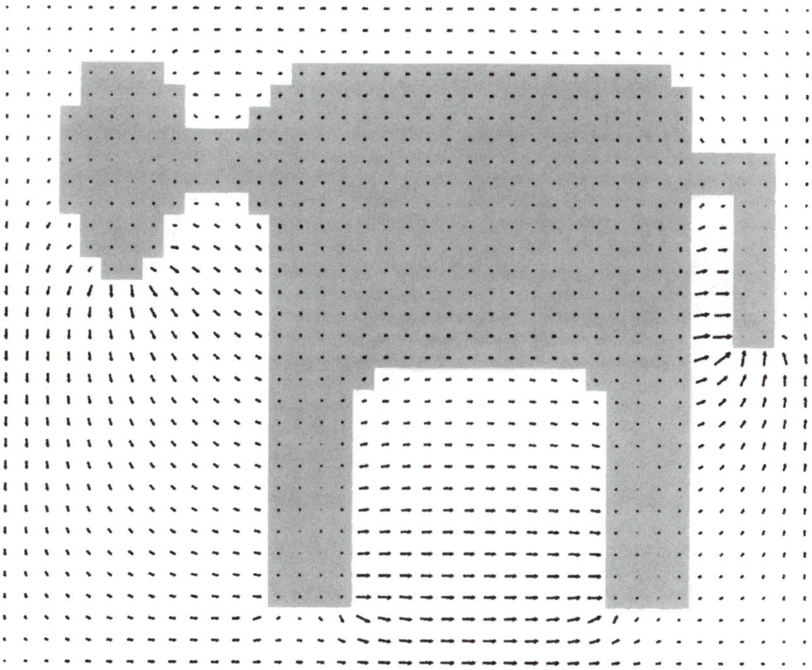

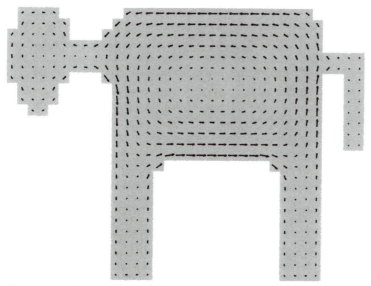

FIGURE 2.32   Calculated **E** fields in a 2D coarse model of an animal in free space exposed to a uniform 60-Hz **B** field in a direction out of the paper. The conductivity of the animal is 0.6 S/m.

FIGURE 2.33   The same model as in Figure 2.32 but showing only the **E** fields inside the animal plotted to a different scale to show the internal fields more clearly.

region of the biological sample. The calculations described below approximate the laboratory **B** fields by spatially uniform **B** fields, which is often a satisfactory approximation.

Calculated **E** fields induced by a spatially uniform, sinusoidally time-varying 60-Hz applied **B** field in a 2D model of a saline solution in a round container with nonconducting walls are shown in Figure 2.37. Consistent with the discussions related to previous examples, the **E** field circulates

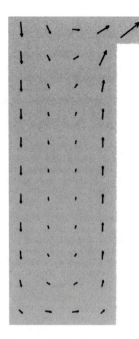

FIGURE 2.34   A view of just the left leg attached to the model of Figure 2.32 and the **E** fields inside it.

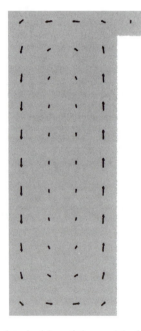

FIGURE 2.35   The **E** fields inside a detached leg of the model of Figure 2.32 plotted to the same scale as those in the attached leg in Figure 2.34.

around the applied **B** field. This is shown more clearly in Figure 2.38, which displays the **E** fields on a coarser grid so that the arrows are longer and the overall pattern is more apparent. On this coarser grid, however, the **E** fields in the wall of the container are no longer identifiable. The square corners in the patterns occur because of the rectangular mathematical grid used to make the calculations. A more realistic pattern would be obtained by using a very large grid and displaying the fields only in the region around the container. This would require more computer memory and

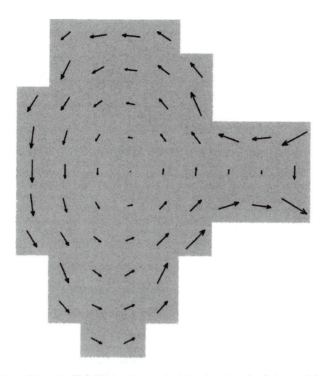

FIGURE 2.36   A view of just the **E** fields in the attached head and neck of the model of Figure 2.33.

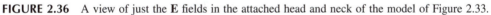

FIGURE 2.37   Calculated **E** fields in a 2D model of a saline solution with a conductivity of 0.6 S/m in a round nonconducting dish exposed to a uniform 60-Hz **B** field in a direction out of the paper.

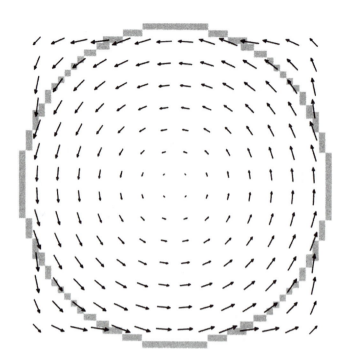

FIGURE 2.38 The **E** fields of Figure 2.37 displayed on a coarser grid to show the field patterns more clearly. Because of the coarser grid, the fields in the wall of the container are not shown specifically.

longer calculation time, but the resulting pattern would be more circularly symmetric, as it would be if the container were in free space.

An interesting question arises about the induced **E**-field pattern if a conducting object were placed in the saline solution of Figure 2.37, such as the round object shown in Figure 2.39. You might expect that the basic pattern of Figure 2.37 would be somewhat modified by the presence of the object but that the pattern in the object would be similar to the pattern in the saline at that position before the object was placed there. To the contrary, however, the close-up view of Figure 2.40 shows that the **E** field inside the conducting object tends to circulate around the object's center, not the center of the dish, as it does in the absence of the object. The center of circulation inside the object is slightly offset, but close to, the center of the object. The fields inside the object are smaller than in the surrounding saline because the conductivity of the object is 8 S/m, while the conductivity of the saline is 0.6 S/m. The presence of the object also changes the pattern in the saline.

Plots of the *currents* in the saline and in the object, as shown in Figures 2.41 and 2.42, give additional insight into the effects caused by the presence of the object. The currents in the object are considerably stronger than in the saline, as shown most clearly in Figure 2.42. Thus, while the higher conductivity of the object causes the **E** fields to be weaker in the object than in the surrounding saline, it also causes the induced currents ($\mathbf{J} = \sigma\mathbf{E}$; see Section 1.6) to be higher in the object than in the surrounding saline. As explained in connection with Figure 1.8, the current pattern inside the object can be thought of as consisting of a global component circulating around the center of the dish and a local component circulating around the center of the object. Because the global component is much the weaker of the two, the combination of the two results in a circulating pattern in the object that is slightly offset from the center of the object.

To illustrate this effect further, the object was placed at the center of the dish, as shown in Figure 2.43. With the object at the center, the global currents and the local currents are one and

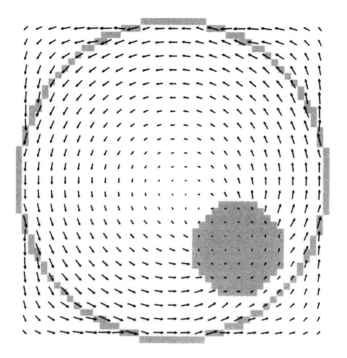

FIGURE 2.39   Calculated **E** fields in the model of Figure 2.37, to which a round object with conductivity of 8 S/m has been added. The fields were calculated on a finer grid and displayed on a coarser grid.

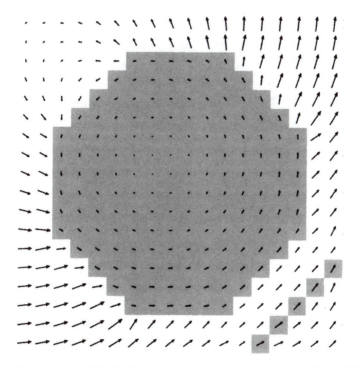

FIGURE 2.40   A close-up view of the field pattern in the region of the object in Figure 2.39, displayed on the finer grid.

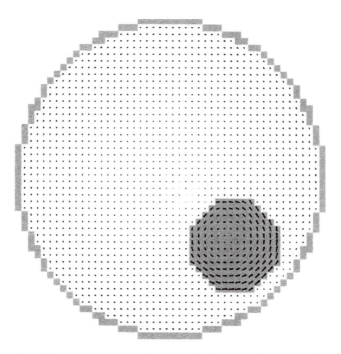

FIGURE 2.41 A plot of the current (conduction plus displacement) in the model of Figure 2.39. The displacement current is negligible, as indicated by the absence of current in the wall of the container.

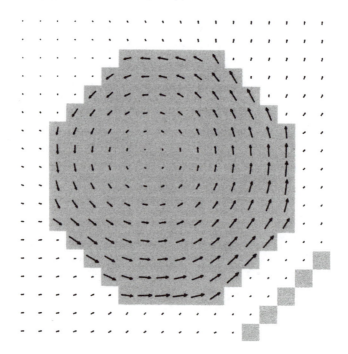

FIGURE 2.42 A close-up view of the currents in the region around the object in Figure 2.41.

the same because they both circulate around the same center. Thus Figure 2.43 shows what the local currents are. Figure 2.44 shows a closer view of these currents. It is apparent that the local currents in Figures 2.42 and 2.44 are nearly the same, which is expected because the conductivity of the object is much greater than that of the saline.

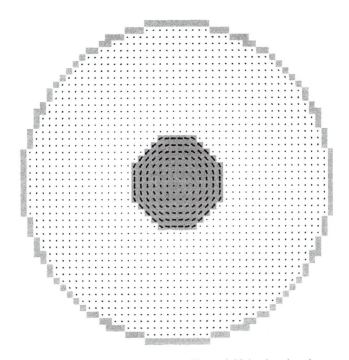

FIGURE 2.43 The current patterns when the object in Figure 2.39 is placed at the center of the dish.

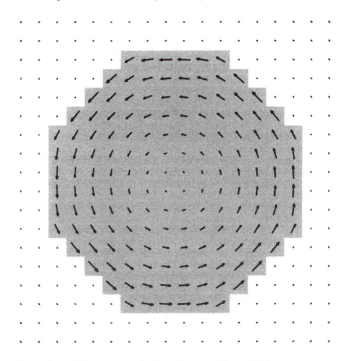

FIGURE 2.44 A closer view of the currents in the object in Figure 2.43.

The behavior illustrated in Figures 2.41 and 2.43 is characteristic of a conducting object placed in a conducting solution exposed to a spatially uniform sinusoidal **B** field. The higher the conductivity of the object compared with the solution, the stronger the local component compared with the global component. This makes the local current pattern less dependent on the exact position of

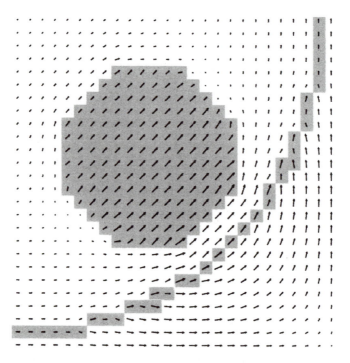

FIGURE 2.45 The **E** fields in the model of Figure 2.39, but with the conducting object changed to a nonconducting dielectric object.

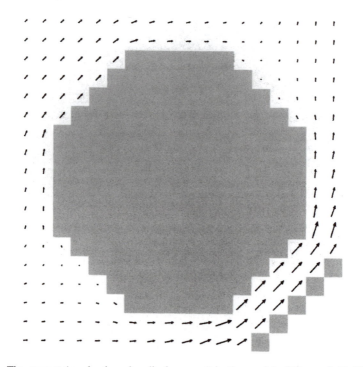

FIGURE 2.46 The current (conduction plus displacement) in the model of Figure 2.45. The displacement current is too small to be visible in the nonconducting object and the nonconducting wall of the container.

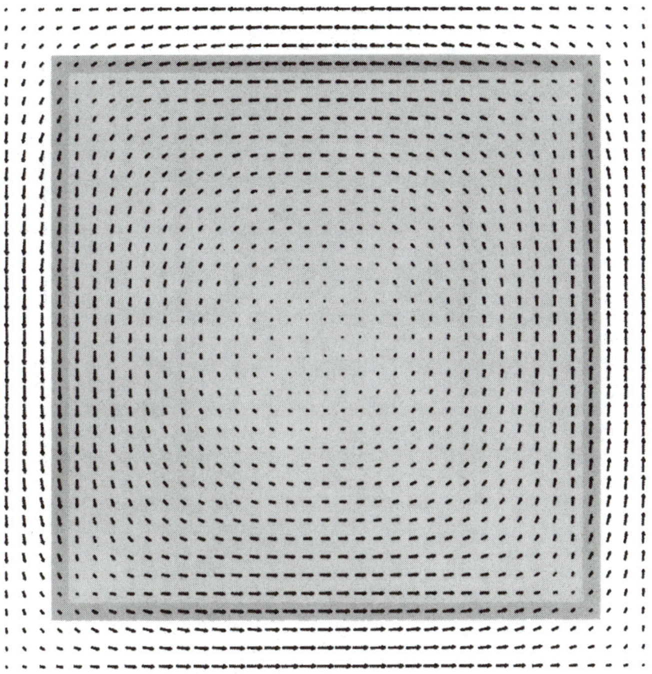

FIGURE 2.47   **E** field induced in a square nonconducting container of saline having a conductivity of 0.6 S/m exposed to a 60-Hz spatially uniform sinusoidal **B** field.

the object within the global pattern. Understanding this behavior is important in designing experiments in which **B** fields are used to expose biological preparations.

A contrasting behavior occurs if the object placed in the solution is nonconducting. The induced **E**-field pattern for this case is shown in Figure 2.45. The **E** fields inside the object are now stronger than those in the surrounding saline. The insulating properties of the object also cause the induced **E** fields to be stronger in the narrow region between the object and the container wall. The plot of the currents shown in Figure 2.46 helps us understand this. The current in the object is negligible because it consists only of displacement current, which is very small because the frequency is so low. Consequently, the current is forced to flow around the object, causing current concentration in the narrow region between the object and the container wall.

What would happen if plate metal electrodes (not connected to any source) were added to a container of conducting solution exposed to a uniform **B** field? To consider this question, first look at Figure 2.47—the **E** fields induced in a square container of saline exposed to a uniform **B** field with no electrodes. The different pattern that results when metal electrodes are added is shown in Figure 2.48, with a close-up view of the upper half shown in Figure 2.49. The electrodes straighten out the **E**-field lines so that in between the electrodes they no longer are circular around the center of the dish. The **E**-field pattern is similar in some respects to the pattern produced by the current source connected between plate electrodes that is shown in Figure 2.23. There is one major difference in the patterns, however. The **E** fields in Figure 2.48 vary approximately linearly with the distance from the horizontal centerline of the dish; note that they are zero along the centerline and even change direction between the top and bottom halves of the electrodes. Except near the ends of the electrodes, they are relatively uniform moving from left to right between the electrodes.

What would the induced **E** fields be in a nonconducting membrane placed in the configuration of Figure 2.48? The results are shown in Figure 2.50, with a close-up view of the membrane in Figure 2.51. The results are very similar to those of Figure 2.26, in which the membrane was placed between electrodes excited by a current source.

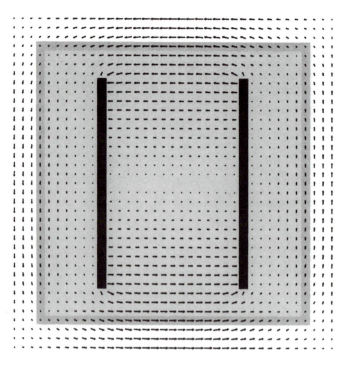

FIGURE 2.48 **E** fields induced in the same configuration as in Figure 2.47 but with plate metal electrodes added. The plates are not connected by any wires.

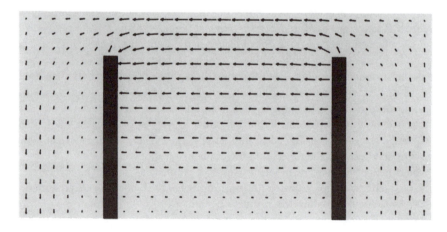

FIGURE 2.49 A close-up view of the upper half of the saline in Figure 2.48.

From the results of this 2D simulation, we might conjecture that metal electrodes in saline exposed to a uniform **B** field could be a good system for *in vitro* exposures to **E** fields if the sample could be placed in a relatively small region up (or down) from the centerline of the dish. This system has an advantage in that it does not require external connections to the metal electrodes, but it does have several disadvantages. The induced **E** field is much less spatially uniform in this system than it is in the system excited by a current source. Furthermore, the magnitude of the **E** fields would be expected to be much smaller for practical values of **B**-field excitation than for practical values of current-source excitation. Careful design would be required to determine whether this kind of **B**-field excitation could be practical.

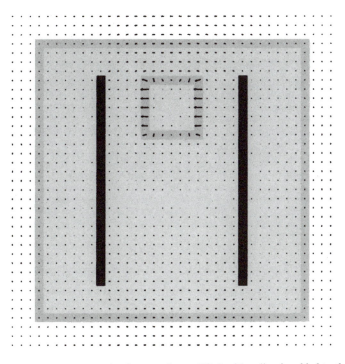

FIGURE 2.50 **E** fields when a nonconducting membrane filled with saline is added to the configuration of Figure 2.48.

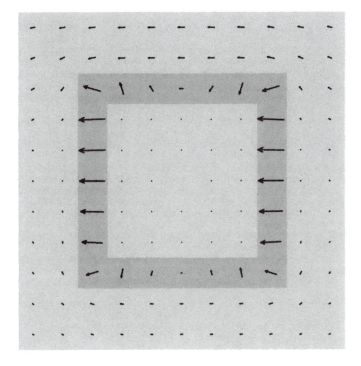

FIGURE 2.51 A close-up view of the **E** fields in and around the membrane of Figure 2.50.

3 EM Behavior When the Wavelength is About the Same Size as the Object

3.1 INTRODUCTION

As explained in Chapter 1, the characteristics of EM fields and their interaction with objects are a strong function of the ratio of the wavelength of the EM fields to object size. Chapter 2 discussed these behaviors when the wavelength was long compared with object size.

This chapter describes and discusses the details of EM field behavior and their interactions when the wavelength is about the same size as the object. According to Figure 1.27, the free-space wavelength is 300 m when the frequency is 1 MHz and is 0.3 mm when the frequency is 1 THz (10^{12} Hz). Consequently, the frequency range addressed in this chapter is approximately between these two frequencies; it is the range designated as "microwave theory" in Figure 1.27.

As explained in Chapter 1, propagation effects dominate in this region of the EM spectrum, and EM field behavior is most often described in terms of wave functions. The wave functions are usually described in terms of $\mathbf{H}$ instead of $\mathbf{B}$ in this range because in the mathematical solution to the equations, it is more convenient to do so. $\mathbf{E}$ and $\mathbf{H}$ are strongly coupled together in this region of the spectrum; one cannot exist without the other. The concept of voltage does not generally apply in this range as it does in the low-frequency range described in Chapter 2, but voltage can be defined in special cases in this range (see Section 3.5.1). Because this chapter deals primarily with waves, their properties, and their interactions with objects, you may wish to review Sections 1.10 and 1.13 before reading it.

3.2 WAVES IN LOSSLESS MEDIA

This section discusses wave properties in terms of two simple waves: spherical waves and plane-waves. Both of these waves are mathematical idealizations. Neither spherical waves nor planewaves exist in perfect form physically, but they are extremely useful for conceptual understanding, and they can approximate real physical waves.

The discussion in this section is restricted to waves propagating in free space and in all space filled with lossless material. Lossless material is material in which the effective conductivity (see Section 1.7) is zero. Wave effects at interfaces between different materials are discussed in Section 3.3, and waves in lossy material are discussed in Section 3.4.

3.2.1 SPHERICAL WAVES

Spherical waves are perhaps the simplest kind of waves to understand. A spherical EM wave consists of an $\mathbf{E}$ field and an $\mathbf{H}$ field that propagate out from a point source. $\mathbf{E}$ and $\mathbf{H}$ are perpendicular to each other, and both are tangent to the surface of an imaginary sphere called a *wavefront*. At any instant of time, the magnitude of $\mathbf{E}$ is the same everywhere on the wavefront. Also, the magnitude of $\mathbf{H}$ is the same everywhere on the wavefront. The direction of propagation of the wave is perpendicular to the spherical wavefront and in a direction radially out from the point source. The vector **k** is often used to describe the direction of propagation of a wave. The relationship between **E**, **H**, and **k** is illustrated in Figure 3.1(a), which shows a cross section of some of the spherical wavefronts and **E**, **H**, and **k** at one point on a wavefront. **E**, **H**, and **k** are mutually perpendicular. If the vector is pointing out of the paper, the tip of the vector is represented by a dot in a circle. If the vector is pointing into the paper, the tail of the vector is represented by a cross in a circle. The vector **k** is in the direction a right-hand screw would move when **E** is turned into **H**. The vector **k** is sometimes called the *ray* of the propagating wave, and the direction of that ray is often a convenient way of describing the path that the electromagnetic energy takes as it propagates through various regions. This is a particularly valuable visualization tool for the case when the wavelength is much smaller than the object. It will be discussed in more detail in Chapter 4.

The characteristics of the wave in the cross section of Figure 3.1(a) can be thought of as similar to the ripples in a pond of water when a pebble is dropped into it. The wave moves out with troughs and crests propagating away from the point at which the pebble entered the water, and the wave eventually dies out by dilution as it gets farther away from the source. Similarly, Figure 3.1(b) shows that the peak magnitude of **E** varies inversely with the radial distance r away from the point source at one instant of time. The magnitude of **H** has a similar variation with r. Figure 3.2 shows how the vectors **E** and **H** vary at one instant of time with distance r along any radial line out from the point source. Figure 3.2 is like a snapshot of **E** and **H**. As time proceeds, the patterns shown in Figure 3.2 move out away from the point source; in other words, the wave propagates.

The ratio E/H is called the *wave impedance*. For spherical waves, the wave impedance is given by

$$Z = \sqrt{\mu/\varepsilon}, \tag{3.1}$$

where μ is the permeability and ε is the permittivity of the medium in which the wave is propagating. For a wave propagating in free space, the wave impedance is 377 Ω (Ω is the symbol for ohms). Since $\varepsilon = \varepsilon_0\varepsilon_r$, where ε_r is the relative permittivity (see Section 1.6), for materials in which $\mu = \mu_0$, the impedance can be written as

$$Z = 377/\sqrt{\varepsilon_r}. \tag{3.2}$$

The velocity of propagation of the wavefronts, called the phase velocity (see Section 1.13), is given by

$$v_p = \frac{1}{\sqrt{\mu\varepsilon}}. \tag{3.3}$$

For a wave propagating in free space, the phase velocity is usually designated by the letter c, and numerically, $c = 1/\sqrt{\mu_0\varepsilon_0} = 3 \times 10^8$ m/s, where μ_0 and ε_0 are the permeability and permittivity, respectively, of free space. As indicated by Equation 3.3, the phase velocity for a wave propagating in a material is lower than c because the permittivity and permeability of any material are greater than those of free space. Thus materials are said to slow down propagating waves. Equation 3.3 can be written for materials in which $\mu = \mu_0$ as

$$v_p = \frac{c}{\sqrt{\varepsilon_r}}. \tag{3.4}$$

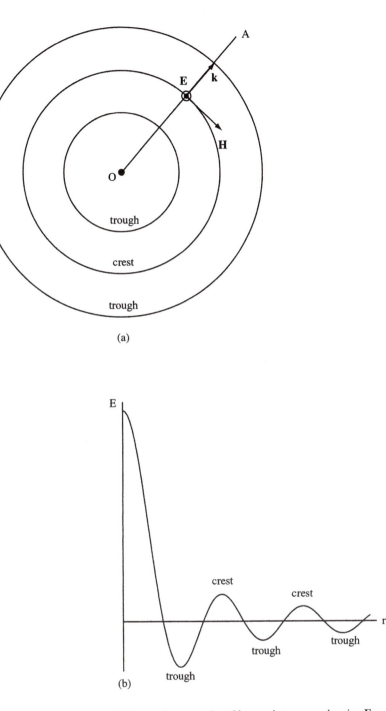

FIGURE 3.1 (a) Cross section of spherical wavefronts produced by a point source, showing **E** and **H** tangent to the wavefront and the propagation vector **k** perpendicular to the wavefront. **E** is directed out of the paper and is therefore represented by a dot in a circle. **E**, **H**, and **k** are mutually perpendicular. (b) The variation of the magnitude of **E** as a function of radial distance r along the line OA at one instant of time. The peak magnitude of **E** varies inversely as r.

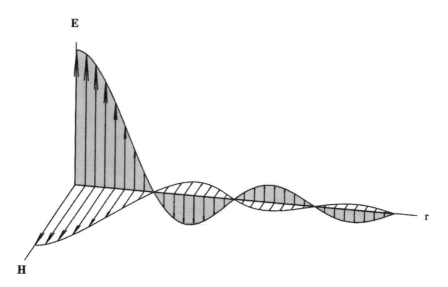

FIGURE 3.2 Pattern showing the **E** and **H** vectors of Figure 3.1 along a radial line at one instant of time. As time progresses, the pattern moves to the right.

For example, if a wave propagates in a material with a relative permittivity of 4, its phase velocity will be half that of a wave propagating in free space.

As mentioned in the introduction to this section, spherical waves do not physically exist; there is no true physical point source of EM fields. The concept of spherical waves is often used to great advantage, however, because it is far simpler both mathematically and conceptually than most physical waves. It is, therefore, used to make calculations for idealized configurations to get approximate results for actual physical configurations. It is also used as a guide in constructing experiments and in interpreting experimental results.

At points far distant from the source in Figure 3.1, the radius of the wavefront is very large, making the curvature of the spherical wavefront so slight that the wavefront is approximately planar in a limited region. This is like the surface of the earth appearing approximately flat to us because the radius of the earth is so large compared with the limited region of our view. When the wavefronts become approximately planar, the wave approximates a *planewave*. This leads us into a discussion of planewaves, which is the subject of the next subsection.

3.2.2 PLANEWAVES

As indicated by the name, planewaves are waves in which the wavefronts are planes. Figure 3.3 illustrates the **E**, **H,** and **k** for a planewave. As for spherical waves, **E**, **H**, and **k** for planewaves are mutually perpendicular, and the direction of **k** is the direction a right-hand screw would move when **E** is turned into **H**. **E** and **H** are tangent to the wavefronts, and **k** is perpendicular to the wavefronts. The magnitude of **E** is the same everywhere on a given planar wavefront. Also, the magnitude of **H** is the same everywhere on a given planar wavefront. Figure 3.4 shows the **E** and **H** patterns at a given instant of time as a function of distance along any line perpendicular to the wavefronts. This figure is like a snapshot of **E** and **H** at a certain instant of time. As time proceeds, the pattern moves to the right. As indicated by Figures 3.3 and 3.4, the magnitudes of **E** and **H** do not decrease with distance in a truly lossless medium. This is unphysical, of course, but true of the idealized planewave.

What kind of source could produce planewaves? Because the **E** and **H** are constant everywhere on a planar wavefront, one would expect that only a source infinite in extent could produce planewaves. Such a source, of course, is unphysical. Perhaps the best approximations to planewaves

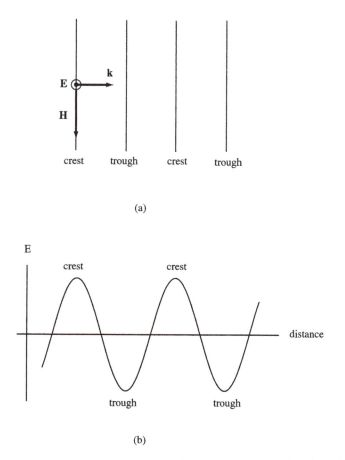

(a)

(b)

FIGURE 3.3 (a) Wavefronts of a planewave. The wavefronts are planes, only the edges of which are shown. **E** and **H** lie within a wavefront. The propagation vector **k** is perpendicular to the wavefronts and points in the direction of propagation. **E**, **H**, and **k** are mutually perpendicular. (b) The variation of the magnitude of **E** at one instant of time as a function of distance perpendicular to the wavefronts.

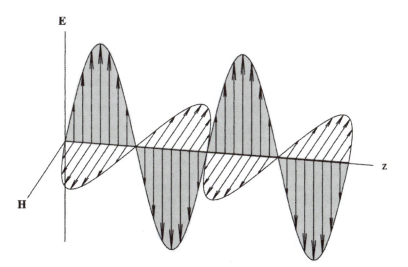

FIGURE 3.4 Pattern showing the **E** and **H** vectors of Figure 3.3 along a line in the direction of **k** at one instant of time. As time progresses, the pattern moves to the right.

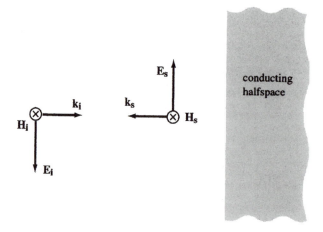

FIGURE 3.5 A planewave normally incident on a planar metallic interface and the reflected planewave produced by the metal. The subscript i stands for the incident wave, and the subscript s stands for the scattered (reflected) wave. The **H** fields are directed into the paper and are therefore represented by a cross in a circle.

are waves produced by very small sources (approximating point sources) when viewed in regions far from the source.

A planewave is similar to a spherical wave in many respects, as you might expect, because a spherical wave approximates a planewave in regions far away from the point source that produces the spherical wave. The wave impedance for a planewave is the same as the wave impedance for a spherical wave, as given by Equation 3.1. The phase velocity for a planewave is the same as the phase velocity for a spherical wave, as given by Equation 3.3. Equation 3.4 also applies to planewaves. A significant difference between planewaves and spherical waves is that the peak magnitudes of the fields in spherical waves vary inversely as distance, while the peak magnitudes of the fields in planewaves remain constant with distance.

If spherical waves and planewaves are unphysical, as we have repeatedly emphasized, why are they used so frequently? Because they are mathematically simple and can be used to understand the basic characteristics of wave interactions, as described in much of the remainder of this chapter.

3.3   WAVE REFLECTION AND REFRACTION

Reflection and *refraction* are two important characteristics of wave behavior. When a propagating wave impinges on an interface between two different materials or on an object, the wave can be reflected, refracted, or both. These behaviors will be illustrated with examples of planewaves impinging on planar interfaces, keeping in mind that planewaves do not exist physically, as explained in the previous section, but that they are extremely useful concepts for explaining important wave characteristics.

3.3.1   PLANEWAVE REFLECTION AT METALLIC INTERFACES

Figure 3.5 illustrates reflection of a planewave that impinges on the interface of a perfectly conducting metallic halfspace (see Section 1.15 for a definition of halfspace). The incident plane-wave is represented by the $\mathbf{E}_i$, $\mathbf{H}_i$, and $\mathbf{k}_i$, which are the electric field, magnetic field, and propagation vector, respectively, of a planewave propagating in free space toward the right. The wave is said to be normally incident on the conducting interface because $\mathbf{k}_i$ is normal to the metallic interface. When the planewave impinges on the metal and begins to propagate into it, the perfect conductivity forces the **E** field to go to zero. The **E** inside the metal must be zero because the conduction current density is given by $\sigma\mathbf{E}$ (σ is conductivity), and since σ is infinite, **E** must be zero, else the conduction

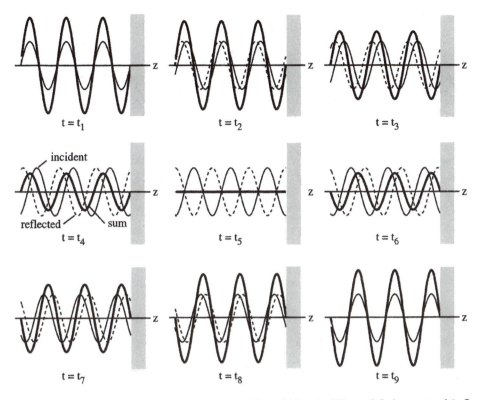

FIGURE 3.6 The electric fields of the incident wave (light solid lines) of Figure 3.5, the scattered (reflected) wave (dashed lines), and the sum of the incident and scattered waves (bold lines) as a function of distance, at nine different instants of time. At t_1 and t_9, the scattered wave lies on top of the incident wave. The gray rectangle represents the position of the planar metallic interface.

current density would be infinite, which is not possible. Because the boundary condition (Equation 1.16) requires the tangential **E** field to be continuous at the metallic interface, and because the **E** field in the metal is zero, the tangential **E** field at the metallic interface must also be zero.

This requirement causes a reflected wave to be generated, with the **E** field of the reflected wave equal and opposite to that of the incident wave at the interface, causing the sum of the two to be zero, thus satisfying the boundary condition. The reflected, or scattered wave, as it is often called, is represented in Figure 3.5 by $\mathbf{E}_s$, $\mathbf{H}_s$, and $\mathbf{k}_s$, which are the electric field, magnetic field, and propagation vector, respectively, of the scattered wave.

The total EM fields in the space to the left of the conducting halfspace in Figure 3.5 are the sums of the incident and scattered fields. Figure 3.6 shows the incident and reflected E-field waves and their sum at nine different instants of time. The sum is zero at the metallic interface for all instants of time. If you look closely at Figure 3.6, you will see that at certain positions in front of the metallic interface, the sum of the incident and reflected waves is zero for all nine instants of time. This is shown more clearly in Figure 3.7(a), which shows just the sum of the incident and reflected wave electric fields as a function of distance z at all nine instants of time superposed on the same graph. At points that lie at half-wavelength intervals back from the metallic surface, the total **E** is zero at all nine instants of time. It turns out that at these points, the **E** is zero at all instants of time, not just the nine shown in the figure. These zero values of **E** are called *nulls*. The nulls occur because the incident and scattered **E** fields are equal in magnitude and opposite in sign at those points so that they cancel each other out at all times. This cancellation occurs because the incident and scattered waves propagate with the same phase velocity, but in opposite directions, and because the incident and scattered **E** must add to zero at the metallic interface.

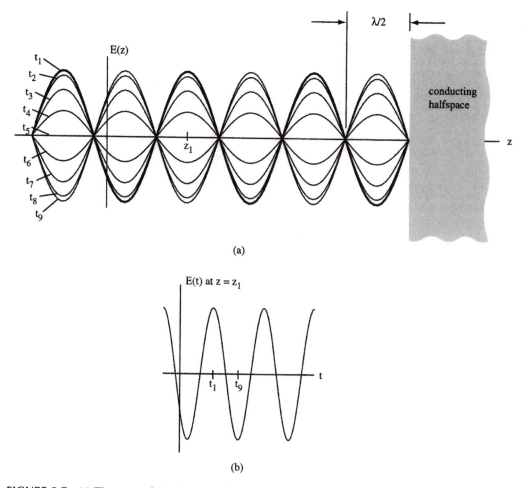

(a)

(b)

FIGURE 3.7   (a) The sums of the electric fields of the incident and scattered waves of Figure 3.6 for nine instants of time all plotted on the same graph as a function of distance in front of the planar metallic object. The E at t_1 is shown in bold to illustrate the typical pattern. (b) The electric field at position z_1 as a function of time.

At each point in space, the amplitude of the **E** is a sinusoidal function of time. Figure 3.7(b) shows the sinusoidal time variation of the amplitude at one point, $z = z_1$. Because of the nulls, the pattern illustrated in Figure 3.7(a) is called a *standing wave*.

Figure 3.8 shows a similar standing-wave pattern for the total **H** fields. Because of the mutually orthogonal relations between **E**, **H**, and **k** in each of the waves, the incident and scattered **H** fields add at the metallic interface instead of canceling, and the first null in **H** occurs a quarter-wavelength back from the metallic interface and then at half-wavelength intervals thereafter.

Standing-wave patterns are often represented by just the *envelope* of the pattern, as shown in Figure 3.9. The envelopes of the **E** and **H** standing waves clearly show the positions of the nulls and the maximum values that the **E** and **H** attain.

Figure 3.10 shows a planewave obliquely incident on a perfectly conducting halfspace. The angle θ_i that the propagation vector ($\mathbf{k}_i$) makes with a normal to the metallic surface is called the *angle of incidence*. As with normal incidence, the boundary conditions at the metallic interface require the tangential electric field to be zero there, thus producing a scattered wave. The angle that $\mathbf{k}_s$ makes with a normal to the surface, θ_s, equals the angle of incidence. Once again, the sum of the electric fields of the incident and scattered waves is a standing wave, but for oblique incidence

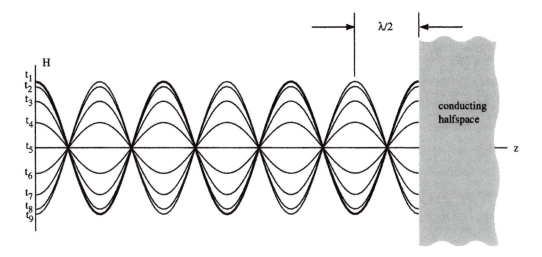

FIGURE 3.8 The sums of the magnetic fields of the incident and scattered waves of Figure 3.6 for nine instants of time all plotted on the same graph as a function of distance in front of the planar metallic object. The H at t_1 is shown in bold to illustrate the typical pattern.

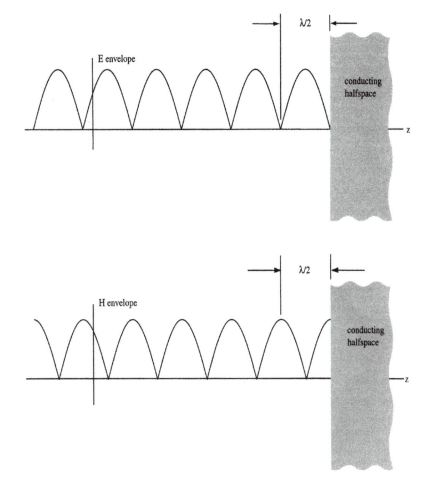

FIGURE 3.9 Envelopes of the **E** and **H** standing waves of Figures 3.7 and 3.8.

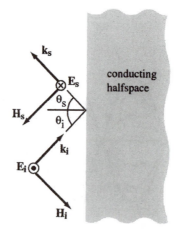

FIGURE 3.10   A planewave obliquely incident on a perfectly conducting planar metallic interface and the reflected (scattered) planewave produced by the metal. The subscript i stands for the incident wave, and the subscript s stands for the scattered (reflected) wave. The angle of reflection θ_s is equal to θ_i, the angle of incidence.

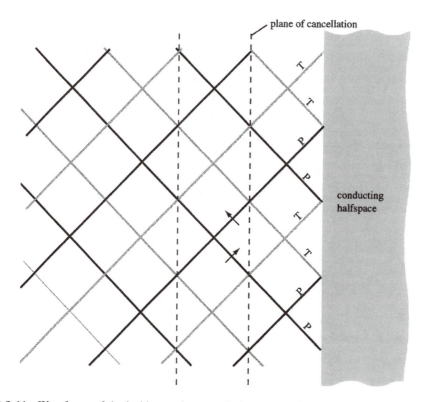

FIGURE 3.11   Wavefronts of the incident and scattered planewaves of Figure 3.10 at one instant of time. P stands for peak, and T stands for trough. The dashed lines show where the peaks and troughs add to zero.

the nulls are farther apart than one-half wavelength. The greater the angle of incidence, the farther apart the nulls.

Figure 3.11 shows the incident and scattered waves at one instant of time in terms of the peaks and troughs—the peaks in black and the troughs in gray. At points where black and gray lines intersect, the sum of the **E** in the two waves is zero. Although intermediate values of **E** between

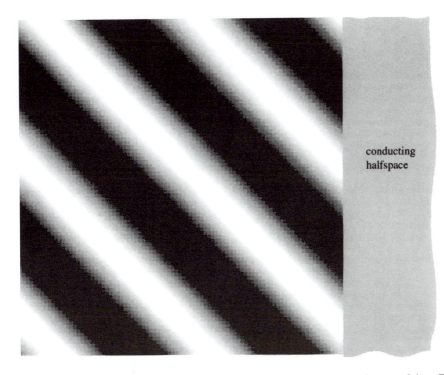

conducting
halfspace

FIGURE 3.12   The amplitude of the **E** of the incident wave of Figure 3.10 at one instant of time. The peaks are white, and the troughs are black. Values in between peaks and troughs are shown in various shades of gray.

the peaks and troughs are not explicitly shown in Figure 3.11, the sum of the incident and scattered **E** is zero everywhere along the dashed lines at every instant of time. Thus a standing wave pattern occurs for oblique incidence just as it does for normal incidence, but the nulls in the standing wave for oblique incidence are farther apart than for normal incidence, as mentioned above.

Another way to illustrate the electric fields of the incident and reflected waves and their sum is shown in Figures 3.12–3.14. In these figures, the amplitude of the **E** is represented by shades of gray, with white showing peaks and black showing troughs. Figure 3.12 shows the **E** of the incident wave at one instant of time, Figure 3.13 the **E** of the scattered wave, and Figure 3.14 the sum of the two. As time progresses, the patterns move according to the propagation properties of the waves, but the nulls in the total **E** always occur at positions corresponding to the dashed lines in Figures 3.11 and 3.14.

3.3.2   PLANEWAVE REFLECTION AND REFRACTION AT DIELECTRIC INTERFACES

As explained in the previous section, perfect conductivity causes the **E** inside a perfect conductor to be zero. And since the boundary conditions require the tangential **E** to be continuous at interfaces, the tangential **E** must be zero at the surface of a perfect conductor. This boundary condition causes a reflected, or scattered, wave to be produced when a wave is incident on a perfect conductor. A reflected wave is also produced when a wave is incident on a good, but not perfect, conductor because the **E** field will be very small, but not zero, in the good conductor. Quite a different effect occurs in a dielectric in which the internal **E** field is not zero. The boundary conditions (Equations 1.15–1.16) at the surface of a dielectric also produce a scattered wave, but in addition, a wave is transmitted into the dielectric.

Figure 3.15 shows a planewave normally incident on a dielectric halfspace, along with the resulting scattered and transmitted waves. The boundary conditions require that the sum of the incident and scattered **E** be equal to the transmitted **E** *at the dielectric interface*. As shown in

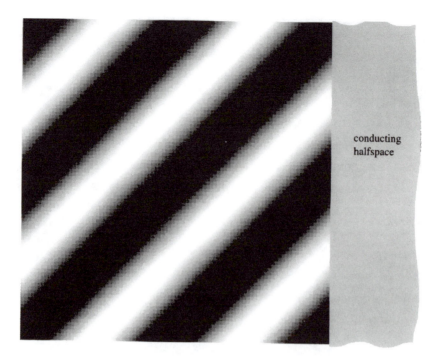

FIGURE 3.13   The amplitude of the **E** of the scattered wave of Figure 3.10 at one instant of time. The peaks are white, and the troughs are black. Values in between peaks and troughs are shown in various shades of gray.

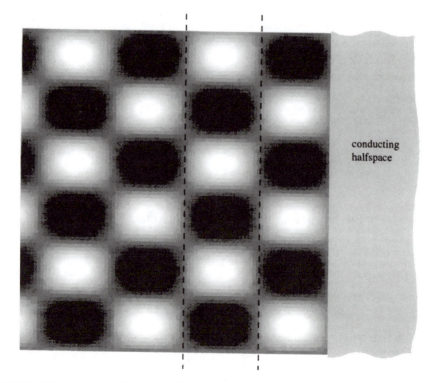

FIGURE 3.14   The amplitude of the sum of the **E** of the incident wave and the **E** of the scattered wave of Figure 3.10 at one instant of time. The peaks are white, and the troughs are black. Values in between the peaks and troughs are shown in various shades of gray. The dashed lines indicate planes of cancellation of the incident and scattered waves.

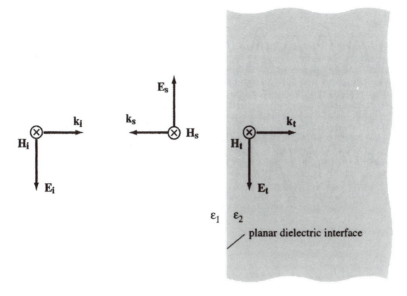

FIGURE 3.15 A planewave normally incident on a planar dielectric interface and the scattered and transmitted planewaves. The subscript i stands for the incident wave, the subscript s stands for the scattered (reflected) wave, and the subscript t stands for the wave transmitted into the dielectric.

Figure 3.16(a) for several instances of time during an oscillatory cycle, the sum of the incident and scattered electric fields in front of the dielectric produces a pattern that is similar to the standing wave in front of the metal (Figure 3.7). But in the pattern produced by the dielectric interface, there are no nulls, just minima. Since there seems to be no standard name for this kind of pattern, in this book it will be called a *wave pattern*. The **E** transmitted into the dielectric is a traveling wave, and its envelope is the same everywhere.

The envelopes of the waves in Figure 3.16(a) are shown in Figure 3.16(b). Because the amplitude of the reflected wave increases and the minima become smaller as the permittivity of the dielectric increases, the wave pattern approaches that of a standing wave for dielectrics of very high permittivity. Also, as the permittivity of the dielectric increases, the amplitude of the transmitted wave decreases. Thus, a high-permittivity dielectric reflects waves similarly to a good conductor.

When a planewave is obliquely incident on a dielectric halfspace (Figure 3.17), the angle of reflection is equal to the angle of incidence, as it is with a conductor (Figure 3.10). The angle of refraction, θ_t, depends on θ_i and the permittivity of the dielectric. For a given θ_i, θ_t decreases as the permittivity increases. The relation between these three quantities is a famous one called *Snell's law of refraction*:

$$\sqrt{\varepsilon_1} \sin \theta_i = \sqrt{\varepsilon_2} \sin \theta_t \tag{3.5}$$

where ε_1 is the permittivity of the dielectric in which the incident and scattered waves propagate, and ε_2 is the permittivity of the dielectric into which the transmitted wave propagates.

When ε_2 is less than ε_1, that is when the incident wave impinges on a medium of lesser permittivity, a special effect called *total internal reflection* can occur. This corresponds to θ_t being equal to or greater than 90°, for which angles the wave would not be transmitted into the second medium. The angle of incidence for which $\theta_t = 90°$ is called the *critical angle*, θ_{ic}. From Equation 3.5 one can solve for θ_{ic} using the fact that when $\theta_t = 90°$, $\sin \theta_t = 1$. Substituting this value in and solving for $\sin \theta_{ic}$ gives

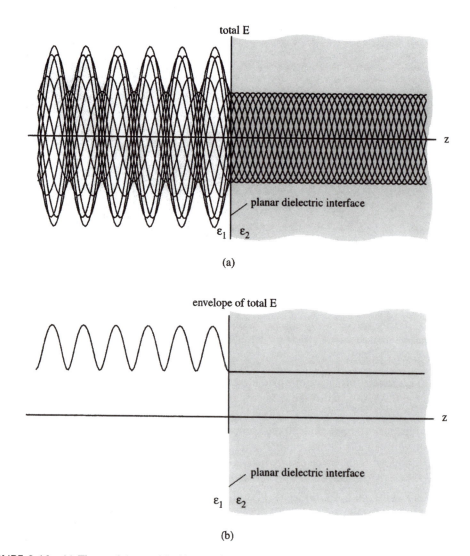

FIGURE 3.16 (a) The total (sum of incident and scattered) $\mathbf{E}$ to the left of the planar dielectric interface and the transmitted $\mathbf{E}$ in the dielectric medium on the right at 13 different instants of time for the waves of Figure 3.15, all plotted on the same graph as a function of distance. $\varepsilon_1 = \varepsilon_0$ and $\varepsilon_2 = 4\varepsilon_0$. (b) Envelope of the $\mathbf{E}$ of (a).

$$\sin \theta_{ic} = \sqrt{\frac{\varepsilon_2}{\varepsilon_1}}. \tag{3.6}$$

For example, if medium 2 is air and medium 1 has a relative permittivity of 4, then $\varepsilon_2/\varepsilon_1 = 1/4$, and $\theta_{ic} = 30°$. Then, as illustrated in Figure 3.18, only waves within a cone of $60°$ would be transmitted out from the dielectric (with reduced amplitude), and all others would be totally internally reflected.

Several important characteristics of wave reflection and refraction by multiple interfaces are illustrated by the simple case shown in Figure 3.19, a planewave propagating to the right and normally incident on a dielectric slab. A dielectric slab is an object that is of a specified thickness in the direction of the $\mathbf{k}_{1a}$ vector in Figure 3.19 and infinite in extent in all other directions. When the wave impinges on the left interface of the slab, part of it is transmitted into the slab and part

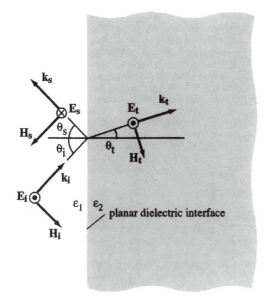

FIGURE 3.17 A planewave obliquely incident on a planar dielectric interface and the scattered and transmitted planewaves. The subscript i stands for the incident wave, the subscript s stands for the scattered (reflected) wave, and the subscript t stands for the wave transmitted into the dielectric.

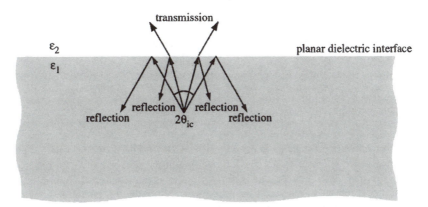

FIGURE 3.18 Waves incident on a lower permittivity medium from a higher permittivity medium at two angles, one less than the critical angle where there is some transmitted portion, and one at the critical angle where there is no longer any wave transmitted into the upper region. If medium 2 is air and medium 1 has a relative permittivity of 4, the critical angle is 30°. For angles of incidence greater than 30°, the waves will not be transmitted into the air but will be totally reflected back into medium 1.

of it is reflected. The part that is transmitted impinges on the right interface, and part of it is transmitted and part is reflected. The part that is reflected travels to the left and impinges on the left interface, where part of it is transmitted and part of it is reflected. This continues until the steady state is reached, which then consists of multiple transmissions and reflections at each interface. In the figure, the subscript a represents the sum of all the waves traveling to the right, and the subscript b represents all those traveling to the left. The combination of all these waves results in a wave pattern similar to those shown in Figure 3.16.

Figure 3.20 shows the electric-field envelopes of these wave patterns as a function of the thickness of a lossless (zero-effective conductivity) dielectric slab having a relative permittivity of 4. The thickness is given in terms of the wavelength inside the dielectric slab, λ_d. Because the

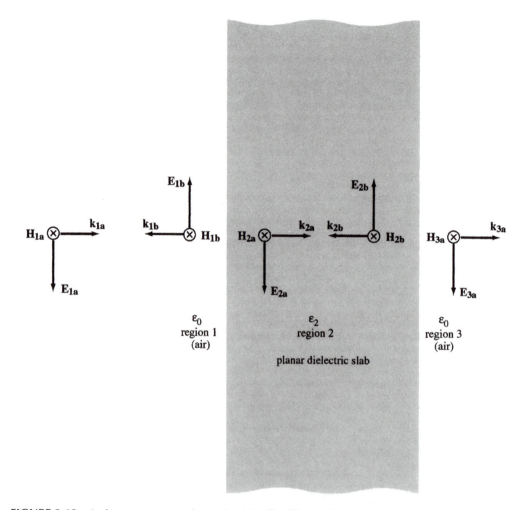

FIGURE 3.19 A planewave propagating to the right ($\mathbf{E}_{1a}$, $\mathbf{H}_{1a}$, $\mathbf{k}_{1a}$) is normally incident on a planar lossless (zero effective conductivity) dielectric slab. The left interface of the slab partially transmits and reflects the planewave. The wave transmitted into the slab is partially transmitted and reflected at the right interface. The wave in the slab that is reflected at the right interface travels left to the left interface and is there partially transmitted and reflected. The process continues until the steady state is reached, which consists of multiple partial transmissions and reflections at each interface. The subscripts a on the $\mathbf{E}$, $\mathbf{H}$, and $\mathbf{k}$ in each region represent the total of all the waves traveling to the right. The subscripts b represent the total of all the waves traveling to the left.

dielectric decreases the velocity of propagation of the planewave according to Equation 3.4, the wavelength in the dielectric, as obtained from Equation 1.25, is given by

$$\lambda_d = \frac{c}{\sqrt{\varepsilon_r} f} = \frac{\lambda}{\sqrt{\varepsilon_r}}, \tag{3.7}$$

where λ is the wavelength in free space ($\lambda = c/f$) and ε_r is the relative permittivity of the dielectric. The dielectric, thus, slows the wave and decreases the wavelength.

As indicated by the graphs in Figure 3.20, the thickness of the slab has a drastic effect on the wave patterns. When the slab is a quarter-wavelength thick, the incident wave is strongly reflected, as indicated by the envelope in Figure 3.20(a) in the free-space region to the left of the slab. The

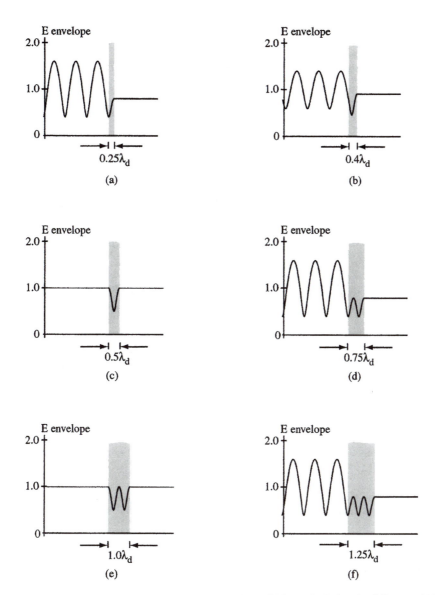

FIGURE 3.20 Electric-field envelopes for the configuration of Figure 3.19 for six different widths of the dielectric slab. The widths are expressed in terms of the wavelength inside the dielectric slab (λ_d). The relative permittivity of each dielectric slab is 4, and the effective conductivity is zero (it is a lossless dielectric).

straight line to the right of each slab represents the envelope of a traveling wave. The height of this envelope indicates how much of the incident wave (which has an envelope of unity height) is transmitted through the slab. As shown in Figure 3.20(a), the transmitted height is less than unity. When the thickness is increased to $0.4\lambda_d$, more of the incident wave is transmitted through the slab, as shown in Figure 3.20(b). When the thickness is increased to one-half a wavelength, a striking effect occurs. All of the incident wave is transmitted through the slab, as shown in Figure 3.20(c). Reflections still occur inside the slab, but no reflections occur at the left interface, as indicated by the flat line to the left of the slab, and the envelope of the transmitted wave to the right of the slab is the same height as that of the incident wave.

As the thickness is increased to $0.75\lambda_d$, strong reflection again occurs. Then for a thickness of one wavelength, all of the incident wave is again transmitted through the slab. Finally, at $1.25\lambda_d$,

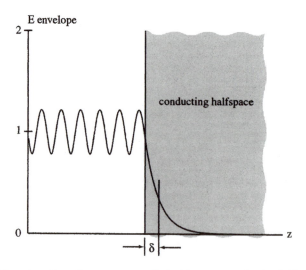

FIGURE 3.21   E-field envelope for a planewave normally incident on a conducting halfspace. δ is the skin depth.

the same reflection occurs to the left as occurs for $0.25\lambda_d$, but multiple maxima and minima occur inside the slab. For multiples of a half wavelength, all of the wave is transmitted through the slab. For odd multiples of a quarter wavelength, strong reflection and low transmission occur.

The characteristics illustrated by Figure 3.20(c) and (e), in which zero reflection and maximum transmission occur, have important practical applications because the same kind of characteristics occur for real waves and nonplanar dielectric objects. For example, dielectric covers (radomes) for radar antennas are made multiples of a half wavelength in thickness to transmit the radar signals through with minimum reflection.

3.4   WAVES IN LOSSY MEDIA

Lossy media are those in which the conductivity, or effective conductivity (see Section 1.7), is not negligible. If the conductivity is high, as it is in metals, the material is called a conductor. If the conductivity is relatively low, the material is called a lossy dielectric. This section first discusses waves in metals and then discusses waves in lossy dielectrics.

3.4.1   WAVES IN METALS

As explained in Section 3.3.1, the **E** inside a perfect conductor (infinite conductivity) must be zero because the conduction current density is given by $\sigma\mathbf{E}$. And since σ is infinite, **E** must be zero or else the conduction current density would be infinite, which is not possible. If the conductivity is high but not infinite, the **E** inside the metal is not forced to be zero, but it is small. As a wave propagates in a good, but not perfect, conductor, the conductivity causes the wave to attenuate because the **E** fields of the wave transfer energy to the charges in the conductor.

Figure 3.21 shows the **E**-field envelope of a planewave impinging normally on a conducting halfspace. As indicated by the envelope, the interface creates a reflected wave that causes a wave pattern to the left of the interface. The conductivity of the halfspace also attenuates the wave as it propagates into the halfspace. We set the conductivity in Figure 3.21 to be relatively low so that the nature of the attenuation is more evident.

When the conductivity is very high, the attenuation is so rapid that the **E** and **H** fields become essentially zero within a very small distance of the interface. The associated currents that flow in the material are therefore confined to a very thin layer near the surface. This effect is called the *skin effect*. The skin depth δ is defined as the depth at which the **E** and **H** have attenuated to $1/e$

(0.37) of their values at the surface (e = 2.718 is the base of the natural logarithm). The skin depth is shown on the diagram in Figure 3.21.

For a planewave impinging on a conducting halfspace, the skin depth is given by

$$\delta = \sqrt{\frac{2}{\omega\mu\sigma}}\,\text{m},\tag{3.8}$$

where ω is the radian frequency, μ is the permeability, and σ is the conductivity. When ω and σ are both high, the skin depth is very small. For example, the conductivity of copper is 5.80×10^7 S/m and the permeability is $4\pi \times 10^{-7}$ H/m. Thus in copper at a frequency of 10 GHz, the skin depth is given by $\delta = \sqrt{2/\left(2\pi 10 \times 10^9 \times 4\pi 10^{-7} \times 5.80 \times 10^7\right)} = 0.66 \times 10^{-6}$ m. The skin depth in other good conductors is similarly very small at high frequencies. At lower frequencies, the skin depth is correspondingly greater, as given by Equation 3.8.

3.4.2 WAVES IN LOSSY DIELECTRICS

The wave pattern for a planewave impinging on a lossy dielectric halfspace is similar to that shown in Figure 3.21 for a conducting halfspace. As mentioned above, conductors are materials having relatively high conductivity and lossy dielectrics are materials having relatively low conductivity. The definition for the skin depth is the same for both kinds of materials. Thus the wave pattern in Figure 3.21 could be for a poor conductor or for a lossy dielectric. The skin depth as a function of frequency for tissue (a lossy dielectric) is shown in Figure 1.29, in which the conductivity is the effective conductivity (see Section 1.7), which varies with frequency.

Wave patterns produced by a lossy dielectric slab are shown in Figure 3.22. Comparison with those of Figure 3.20 for the lossless slab show that the loss has a significant effect on the wave patterns. The envelopes inside the slab show how the loss decreases the amplitudes of the waves as they travel through the slab. A particularly significant effect of the loss is that zero reflection no longer occurs when the thickness of the slab is a multiple of a half wavelength, as indicated by the patterns of Figure 3.21(c) and (e).

3.4.3 ENERGY ABSORPTION IN LOSSY MEDIA

The *Poynting vector* describes the density of the time rate of change of the energy (the power) stored in the **E** and **H** fields in a wave. For sinusoidal planewaves, the magnitude of the time-average Poynting vector is given by

$$P = \sqrt{\frac{\varepsilon}{\mu}}E_{\text{rms}}^2 \ \text{W}/\text{m}^2\tag{3.9}$$

in terms of the **E** of the planewave, or equivalently by

$$P = \sqrt{\frac{\mu}{\varepsilon}}H_{\text{rms}}^2 \ \text{W}/\text{m}^2\tag{3.10}$$

in terms of the **H** of the planewave. The Poynting vector may be thought of as describing the power per unit area that can be transferred to the material in which the wave is propagating. These two relations are used in dosimetry (see Chapter 5) in relating the energy absorbed in models of humans and other animals to the fields and power of the incident waves.

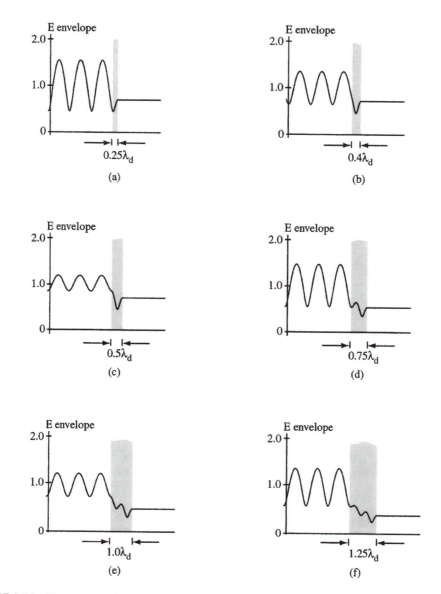

FIGURE 3.22 The same graphs as in Figure 3.20, but for this case the dielectric is lossy.

The SAR (see Section 1.7) that describes the time rate of energy transferred from a planewave to a material (per unit mass) at a given point is given by Equation 1.11. Because the envelope of E is the peak value of the **E** field at each point, and since the rms value is equal to 1/2 the peak value (see Section 1.12), the SAR is proportional to the square of the envelope. Thus the envelopes inside the dielectric slabs of Figure 3.22 indicate that the SARs can vary significantly from point to point inside the slabs.

Figure 3.23 shows examples of the SAR inside lossy dielectric slabs. Figure 3.24 shows the same information in terms of a gray-scale plot on a larger scale. The gray-scale display dramatizes the strong variation of the SAR with position in the slab (maximum SAR is shown as white and minimum is shown as black). The brighter areas are near the left sides of the slabs, where the EM wave is incident, and the darker areas are toward the right side of the slabs, where the EM wave has been attenuated by the losses in the slabs. The SAR pattern is a strong function of the thickness of the slab compared with the wavelength of the EM radiation.

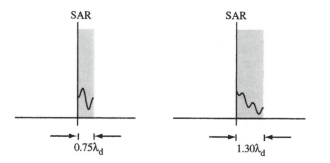

FIGURE 3.23 SAR distributions in lossy dielectric slabs similar to those in Figure 3.22.

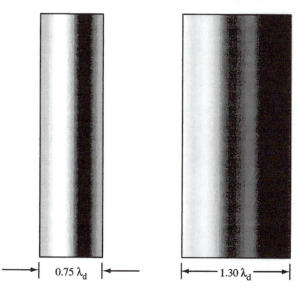

FIGURE 3.24 The SAR distributions in the lossy slabs of Figure 3.23 shown as gray-scale distributions. Maximum SAR is shown as white, and minimum is shown as black.

The bright areas are often referred to as "hot spots," although this is not precise nomenclature because "hot" refers to temperature, and temperature inside a body exposed to EM radiation depends not only on the SAR but also on the thermal properties of the body. For example,in animals, the temperature is a strong function of the thermal regulatory mechanisms of the body, such as increased blood perfusion.

These examples illustrate the general characteristics of SAR distributions inside the bodies of humans and other animals exposed to EM radiation. The distribution inside the body is a strong function of the size of the body compared with the wavelength of the EM radiation, and when the body size is of the same order of magnitude as the wavelength, the SAR distribution is usually very nonuniform. The nonuniformity is caused by the multiple reflections and refractions at the interfaces between materials of different electrical properties. While the examples given here are for homogeneous slabs, the nonuniformities are further increased by inhomogeneities in objects, like the inhomogeneous tissues of animal bodies.

3.5 TRANSMISSION LINES AND WAVEGUIDES

The sections above discussed free-space wave propagation, reflection, and refraction. This section describes wave propagation along guiding systems (transmission systems), such as two-wire transmission lines, coaxial cables, and hollow pipes called waveguides. Such systems are widely used to transmit EM signals when the frequency is high enough that the wavelength of the EM fields is of the same order of magnitude as the size of the transmission system.

When waves propagate along guiding systems, the **E** fields and **H** fields exist in characteristic combinations called *modes*. The three most common modes are transverse electromagnetic (TEM), transverse electric (TE), and transverse magnetic (TM). In the TEM mode, both **E** and **H** are transverse (perpendicular) to the direction of propagation. In the TE mode, **E** is transverse, or perpendicular, to the direction of propagation, but **H** is not. In the TM mode, **H** is transverse to the direction of propagation, but **E** is not. A planewave, for example, is a TEM wave because, as explained in Section 3.2.2, **E** and **H** are both perpendicular to the propagation vector **k**, which lies along the direction of propagation.

TEM modes can exist on structures consisting of two conductors, such as two wires or a coaxial cable, which consists of a wire centered inside a hollow pipe, but they cannot exist in hollow pipes. This section first discusses TEM transmission systems, which are usually referred to as transmission lines, and then discusses waveguides, which propagate combinations of TE and TM modes.

3.5.1 TEM Systems

Section 1.14 states that when the frequency is high enough that the wavelength is comparable to the size of the system, voltage can be defined only in very special cases. One of those special cases is TEM modes. As explained in Section 1.2, a unique voltage can be defined between two points when **E** is a conservative field. From Equation 1.3, it can be shown that when **E** and **H** lie in the same plane, as they do in TEM modes, that **E** is conservative. Therefore, voltage can be uniquely defined for TEM modes.

TEM modes can exist on transmission systems consisting of two conductors. Several examples of such systems are shown in Figure 3.25. In each case, a source, such as a voltage source or current source, produces a voltage difference between the two conductors and causes current to flow in the conductors. Other modes can also exist on these transmission systems, but when these systems are used, they are usually designed so that the TEM mode dominates and the other modes are negligible.

Figure 3.26 shows the **E**-field pattern at one instant of time between the conductors of the stripline of Figure 3.25(c). A unique potential difference exists between the two conductors because the same amount of work is required to move a charge from one conductor to the other along any path between the two (see Section 1.2). The same is true for all TEM systems. Since a unique potential difference can be defined for TEM transmission systems, transmission along them is usually described in terms of voltage $V(z)$ between the conductors and current $I(z)$ in the conductors (Figure 3.27), each described as a propagating wave. These propagating voltage and current waves on all TEM systems are described by the same set of equations, which are called the transmission-line equations. Thus the characteristic behaviors that result from the solution of these transmission-line equations apply to all TEM systems.

A typical transmission-line configuration is a source applied at the left end of the transmission line, which causes voltage and current waves to propagate along the line, usually to carry information of some kind (a signal) or to transmit energy to some device or system (often called the load, which is represented as a load impedance Z_L). This configuration is diagrammed in Figure 3.28. The source is often a sinusoidal function of time, although it could be any function of time. When it is a sinusoidal function of time, the phasor transform (see Section 1.11) is usually used to solve for the voltages and currents.

The source generates a voltage wave and a current wave that propagate to the right. If the transmission line were infinitely long (a physical impossibility, but a useful concept), only waves traveling to the right would exist. When the line is finite, any kind of discontinuity in the line, such as a change in the size and shape of the conductors, a change in the dielectric properties between

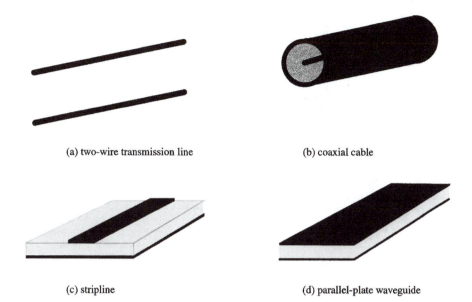

(a) two-wire transmission line (b) coaxial cable

(c) stripline (d) parallel-plate waveguide

FIGURE 3.25 Examples of two-conductor transmission systems. In each case, the conductor is shown in black, and some kind of dielectric material (could be air) is placed between the conductors.

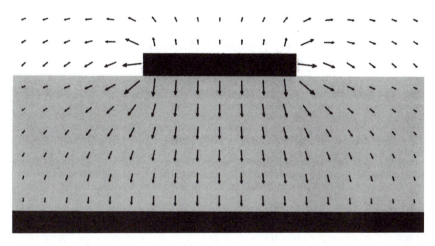

FIGURE 3.26 Two-dimensional calculations of the **E**-field pattern between the two conductors of the stripline shown in Figure 3.25(c). A sinusoidal current source (not shown) is connected between the two conductors. The **E** fields are shown at an instant of time when the source current is zero. The **E** fields are negligibly small at an instant of time when the source current is maximum. This corresponds to a 90° phase shift between the **E** fields and the source current. For clarity, only the central region of the stripline is shown. The fields to the left and to the right of the region shown are very small.

the conductors, or some device connected between the conductors, will cause reflections, that is, waves traveling to the left. These reflections are like those described for planewaves (Section 3.3).

The ratio of the phasor voltage (the sum of the phasor voltage wave traveling to the right and the one traveling to the left) to the phasor current (the sum of the phasor current wave traveling to the right and the one traveling to the left) at any point on the line is called the *impedance*. In general, the impedance is a function of position along the transmission system; that is, it varies with position. When only waves traveling to the right (or to the left, but not both) exist, such as in an infinitely long line, the ratio of the voltage to the current has the same value at any point on

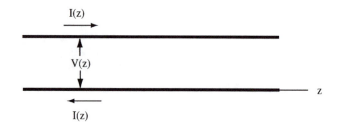

FIGURE 3.27 Voltage and current on a two-wire transmission line. V (z) is the potential difference of one wire with respect to the other at a point z on the transmission line. I (z) is the current in the wire at the point z, with equal and opposite currents in the two wires at that point on the line.

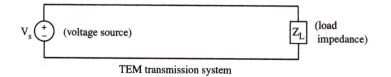

FIGURE 3.28 A diagram of a TEM transmission system with a source (voltage source shown here) connected to the left end and a system or device (represented by a load impedance) connected to the right end. A current source is another typical source that could be connected to a transmission system.

the transmission system. This ratio is called the *characteristic impedance* of the transmission system. The characteristic impedance is usually designated by the symbol Z_0. The characteristic impedance is used to identify and classify important characteristics of the transmission system. For example, typical characteristic impedances of coaxial cable are 50Ω, 75Ω, and 25Ω (Ω stands for ohms). For two-wire transmission lines, such as TV twin lead, Z_0 is typically 300Ω.

The load impedance has a significant effect on the waves traveling on the transmission system, as illustrated in Figure 3.29, which shows envelopes of the voltage along the transmission system for the configuration of Figure 3.28 for various values of load impedance. A short circuit (perfect conductor connected between the two conductors of the transmission system so $Z_L = 0$ as shown in Figure 3.29(a)) causes a standing wave along the line, exactly like the one in Figure 3.9 for the **E** field of a planewave normally incident on a perfect conductor. An open circuit (zero conductivity between the two conductors so $Z_L \rightarrow \infty$ as shown in Figure 3.29(b)) likewise causes a standing wave, but one that is shifted. Other values cause a wave pattern, but not a standing wave because the minima are not nulls.

An especially interesting situation occurs when $Z_L = Z_0$. For this case, there is no reflected wave, and only a wave traveling to the right exists, as indicated by the envelope in Figure 3.29(c), which is a flat line. When $Z_L = Z_0$, the line is terminated in its characteristic impedance, and the line is said to be "flat" (because the envelope is a flat line). The line is also said to be "impedance matched" because the load impedance is equal to the characteristic impedance, or is "matched." In cases where a signal or power is to be transmitted to a load, reflections are usually undesirable, and it is usually better to have a matched line.

Two parameters are defined to describe how well a load is matched to a line. One is the magnitude of the reflection coefficient $|\rho|$ which is defined as

$$|\rho| = \frac{|V_{ref}|}{|V_{inc}|} \tag{3.11}$$

where $|V_{ref}|$ is the magnitude of the voltage wave traveling to the left (the reflected wave) and $|V_{inc}|$ is the magnitude of the voltage wave traveling to the right (the incident wave). When $Z_L = 0$,

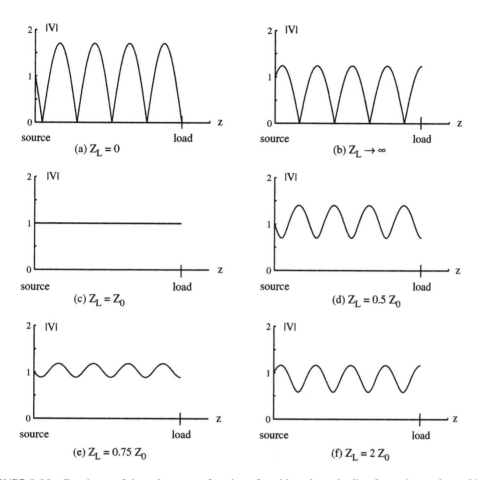

FIGURE 3.29 Envelopes of the voltage as a function of position along the line for various values of load impedance Z_L for the system shown in Figure 3.28. $|V|$ stands for the envelope of V. The voltage source has a magnitude of one volt. $Z_L = 0$ is equivalent to a short circuit, and $Z_L \rightarrow \infty$ is equivalent to an open circuit.

the reflected wave is zero, and $|\rho| = 0$. When $Z_L = 0$, $|\rho| = 1$. Also, when Z_L approaches infinity, $|\rho| = 1$.

The second parameter is the voltage standing wave ratio (VSWR), which is defined as

$$VSWR = \frac{|V|_{max}}{|V|_{min}} \tag{3.12}$$

as illustrated in Figure 3.30. In terms of the reflection coefficient, the VWSR is given by

$$VSWR = \frac{1 + |\rho|}{1 - |\rho|} \tag{3.13}$$

Thus, when $|\rho| = 1$, the VSWR approaches infinity, and when $|\rho| = 0$, the VSWR = 1. This is consistent with the definition in Equation 3.12 because when $|\rho| = 1$, $|V|_{min} = 0$ (as in Figure 3.29(a)), and when $|\rho| = 0$, $|V|_{min} = |V|_{max}$ (as in Figure 3.29(c)). Thus in a matched line, the VSWR = 1.

Reflections are also produced when transmission lines of different characteristic impedances are connected together. For example, if two striplines having different dielectrics between the two

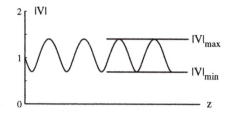

FIGURE 3.30 The maximum and the minimum of the voltage envelope used in defining VSWR.

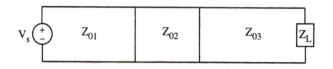

FIGURE 3.31 A diagram of three TEM transmission systems, each having a different characteristic impedance and a different length, connected together. A voltage source is at the left end of the combination, and a
load impedance is connected to the right end.

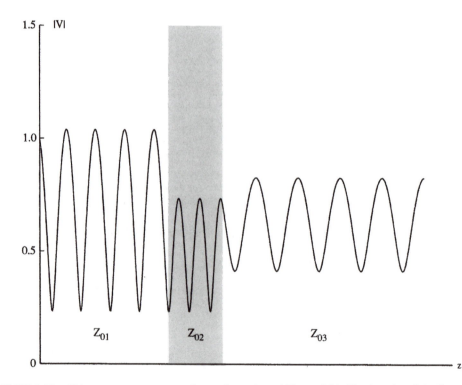

FIGURE 3.32 Voltage wave patterns on the configuration of Figure 3.31. The lengths of the lines are 2.2,
1.3, and 2.4 line wavelengths, respectively. $Z_L = 2 Z_{03}$. $Z_{02} = Z_{01}/\sqrt{2}$. $Z_{03} = \sqrt{2} Z_{01}$.

conductors were connected together, the discontinuity in the dielectrics would produce reflections.
Figure 3.31 shows a diagram representing the connection of three different transmission systems
with different characteristic impedances. The resulting voltage wave patterns for one set of characteristic impedances are shown in Figure 3.32. In general, the voltage wave patterns are a strong
function of the relative characteristic impedances and the lengths of the lines.

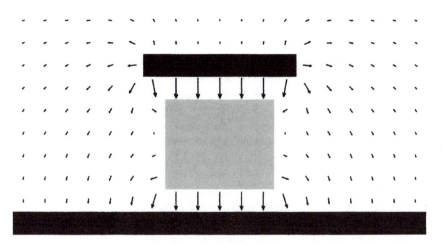

FIGURE 3.33 Two-dimensional simulation of the **E**-field pattern when a biological sample is placed between the conductors of the stripline of Figure 3.26 when the conductors are suspended in air. The conductivity and relative permittivity of the biological sample are 0.4 S/m and 100, respectively. The frequency is 10 MHz. The mathematical cells are 1 mm square. The pattern is for an instant of time when the sinusoidal source current is zero.

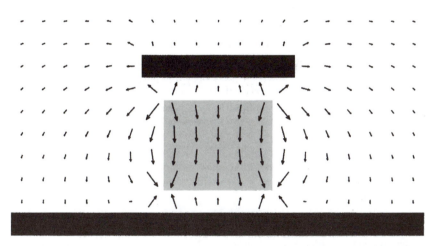

FIGURE 3.34 Same **E**-field pattern as in Figure 3.33 except that it is at an instant of time when the sinusoidal source current is maximum. The plotting scale of this figure is about 400 times greater than in Figure 3.33; that is, the fields in this figure are about 400 times weaker than those in Figure 3.33.

3.5.2 TEM SYSTEMS FOR EXPOSING BIOLOGICAL SAMPLES

Some TEM systems, such as the stripline and the parallel-plate waveguide (Figure 3.25) are sometimes used for exposing biological samples to **E** and **H** fields. Usually, the exposure system is designed to produce the most uniform **E** fields possible throughout the biological sample. As shown by the **E**-field pattern in Figure 3.26 for the stripline, when the dielectric between the conductors is uniform, there is a region in which the **E** field is relatively uniform in a given cross section of the line.

However, if the stripline is suspended in air and a biological sample is placed between the conductors, the **E**-field pattern is modified by the presence of the sample. Figures 3.33 and 3.34 show such patterns for two different instants of time. In Figure 3.33, the **E** fields inside the sample at an instant of time when the source current is zero are negligibly small, and the fields in the surrounding air are relatively very strong. In Figure 3.34, the fields inside and outside the sample are of the same order of magnitude at an instant of time when the source current is maximum, but they are about 400 times smaller than those in Figure 3.33. These two plots together indicate that the **E** fields outside the sample are almost 90° out of phase with the current source, as in a capacitor, and the **E** fields inside the sample are nearly in phase with the current source, as in a resistor.

In addition to the nonuniformities introduced in the cross-sectional variation of the fields in a biological sample placed in a transmission system, nonuniformities in the direction of propagation also pose a problem when uniform exposure throughout the volume of a biological sample is desired. This problem is illustrated by the examples shown in Figures 3.35 and 3.36. Figure 3.35 shows the voltage wave pattern for the configuration of Figure 3.31 in which the middle characteristic impedance represents the presence of the sample in the transmission system. The variation of |V| with respect to z is directly proportional to the variation of E with respect to z. The length of line 3 and Z_L were chosen so that the |V| in the sample is uniform in the z direction. Theoretically, it is usually possible to do this, but practically, small deviations in the frequency or in the transmission-line dimensions due to temperature changes could upset this balance and cause the |V| in the sample not to be uniform in the z direction.

A more serious limitation is illustrated by the pattern in Figure 3.36, which shows what happens when the biological sample is lossy, as it usually is. The loss in the sample causes |V| to decrease with z. This effect can be minimized to some extent by making the sample as short as possible, but it cannot be entirely eliminated.

Because the **E** fields inside the sample are generally not spatially uniform, and because they are much smaller than those in the surrounding air, careful dosimetry must be carried out to interpret the results of experiments that attempt to relate biological effects to applied **E** fields. Another important consideration is that the simulations described above are based on the existence of the TEM mode alone in a two-dimensional model. At higher frequencies, depending on the size and shape of the sample, other modes can exist simultaneously. The presence of other modes could cause the **E** fields to be more spatially nonuniform than the examples above indicate.

3.5.3 WAVEGUIDES

TE and TM systems are generally called *waveguides*. The most common waveguides are hollow rectangular and cylindrical pipes (Figure 3.37) made of highly conducting material fabricated to close dimensional tolerances.

An electromagnetic source, such as a solid-state microwave oscillator or an electron-beam microwave tube, e.g., a klystron or backward-wave oscillator, is often connected to one end of the waveguide, which produces EM waves that propagate down the waveguide. The other end of the waveguide might be connected to a radar antenna, such as a dish, to transmit signals into space. Or, a microwave receiving antenna might be connected to one end of the waveguide and the waveguide used to transmit the received signal to a microwave receiver connected to its other end.

Waveguides are also used to expose biological samples to EM fields. When biological samples are inserted into waveguides, the same considerations with respect to uniformity of the **E** and **H** fields inside the sample occur as with the TEM systems, as described in Section 3.5.2.

To illustrate the concepts of TE and TM modes and their propagation in waveguides, these modes in rectangular waveguides will be discussed in detail. Similar properties and characteristics apply to other kinds of waveguides, such as cylindrical waveguides.

3.5.3.1 TE and TM Mode Patterns in Rectangular Waveguides

An infinite number of TE and TM modes can exist in a rectangular waveguide. Each one consists of a characteristic combination of **E** and **H** field distributions. These modes are designated as TE_{mn} and TM_{mn} modes, where m and n are digits that identify each of the modes. In general, an infinite

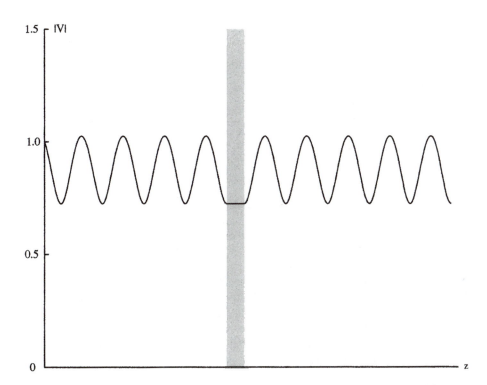

FIGURE 3.35 Voltage wave patterns when the middle characteristic impedance of Figure 3.31 represents a biological sample placed in a TEM transmission system.

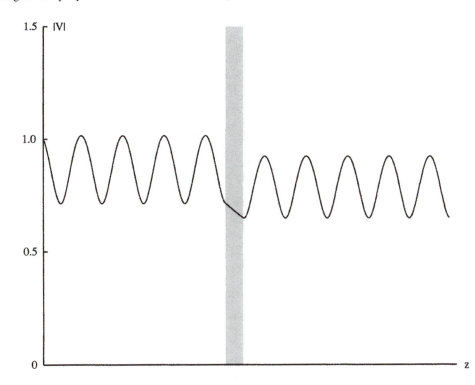

FIGURE 3.36 The same as Figure 3.35 except that the biological sample is lossy.

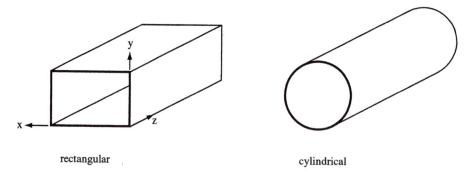

rectangular   cylindrical

FIGURE 3.37   Two commonly used waveguides: rectangular and cylindrical.

number of these TE and TM modes can be present simultaneously in a waveguide, depending on the method of excitation, the size and shape of the waveguide, and the frequency of the waves, as will be explained later. The m specifies how many peaks occur in the mode pattern across the width of the waveguide (the x direction in Figure 3.37), and the n specifies how many peaks occur in the mode pattern across the height of the waveguide (the y direction in Figure 3.37).

Figure 3.38 shows the **E** and **H** vector field patterns at one instant of time for the TE_{10} mode, in which m = 1 and n = 0. The pattern propagates down the waveguide as time goes on. m = 1 indicates that there is one peak across the waveguide. This corresponds to the E_y (the component of **E** in the y direction) having a maximum in the center and being zero on each side wall. Note that in all cases, the boundary conditions (see Section 1.11) require that the tangential component of the **E** field be zero at the metallic walls (assuming that they are perfectly conducting) of the waveguide. In other words, the **E** field must be normal to the perfectly conducting walls. Because E_y is tangential to the side walls, it must be zero there, but because it is normal to the top and bottom walls, it need not be zero there.

n = 0 indicates that there is no variation in the y direction; that is, at a given value of x, all three vectors shown in the diagram have the same length. As another example, mode patterns for the TE_{20} mode are shown in Figure 3.39. Again, there is no variation in the y direction, but m = 2 indicates that two peaks occur across the waveguide. In this case, E_y is zero in the center as well as at the two side walls.

The peaks in the mode patterns are more clearly displayed in terms of the envelopes (see discussion in connection with Figure 3.9 in Section 3.3.1) of **E**, as shown in Figure 3.40 for three modes, TE_{10}, TE_{20}, and TE_{11}. The TE_{10} mode has one peak across the waveguide, and the TE_{20} mode has two peaks across the waveguide. The TE_{11} mode pattern is more complicated than the other two in Figure 3.40 because in it there is one peak across the guide in both the x direction and the y direction, as shown in Figure 3.40(c). Again, the **E** fields are normal to the metallic walls at the walls.

These examples illustrate the nature of mode patterns. Other patterns in rectangular waveguide are similar in nature and behavior. Mode patterns in other kinds of waveguide, such as cylindrical waveguide, are similar in characteristic behavior but differ in detail because of the round shape of the waveguide.

3.5.3.2   Mode Excitation and Cutoff Frequencies

Waveguides are typically excited by a microwave generator, such as an electron-beam tube like a magnetron or a solid-state device like a transistor oscillator that is connected to the waveguide by a coaxial cable. The coaxial cable is typically connected to the waveguide by extending the center conductor of the cable through the top waveguide wall to form a "probe" in the waveguide and connecting the outer conductor of the cable to the waveguide wall, as shown diagrammatically in

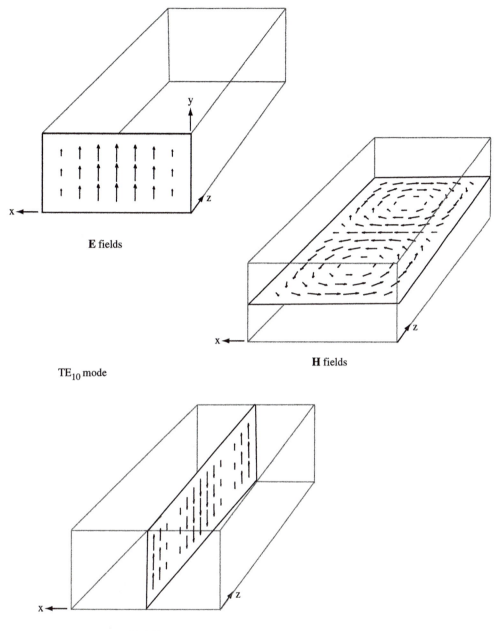

FIGURE 3.38   The TE$_{10}$ mode patterns in three different planes in a rectangular waveguide at one instant of time. As time progresses, the patterns move in the +z direction.

Figure 3.41. The center wire of the coaxial cable can also be formed into a loop and connected back to the waveguide wall to produce "loop" excitation. To excite the TE$_{10}$ mode, the coaxial cable is usually put in the side wall of the waveguide so that the plane of the loop is perpendicular to the **H** fields. The probe, or whatever other method of introducing the microwave fields into the waveguide is used, excites many TE and TM modes that exist simultaneously in the waveguide. Some of these modes propagate, however, and some die away very rapidly from the probe. The modes that die away are called *evanescent* modes.

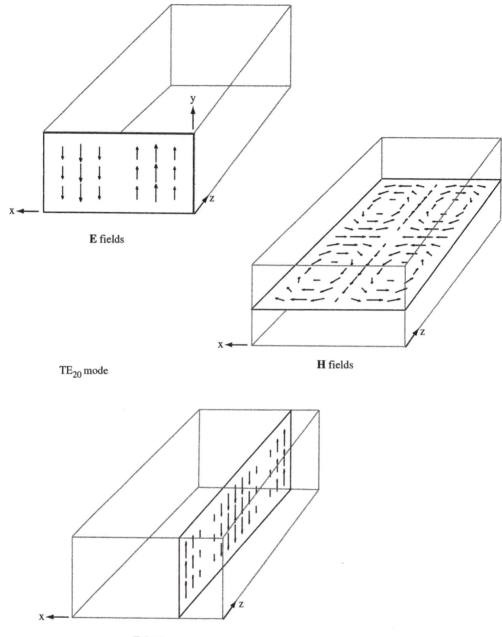

FIGURE 3.39   The TE_{20} mode patterns in three different planes in a rectangular waveguide at one instant of time. As time progresses, the patterns move in the +z direction.

Whether a mode propagates or is evanescent is determined by the frequency of the exciting fields and the size and shape of the waveguide. For each mode, there is a frequency, called the *cutoff frequency* (usually designated by f_{co}) below which the mode will be evanescent and above which the mode will be propagating. The cutoff frequency for each mode depends on the size and shape of the waveguide. For a rectangular waveguide, the TE_{10} mode has the lowest cutoff frequency. Figure 3.42 shows a diagram of how the cutoff frequencies of the various modes are related when

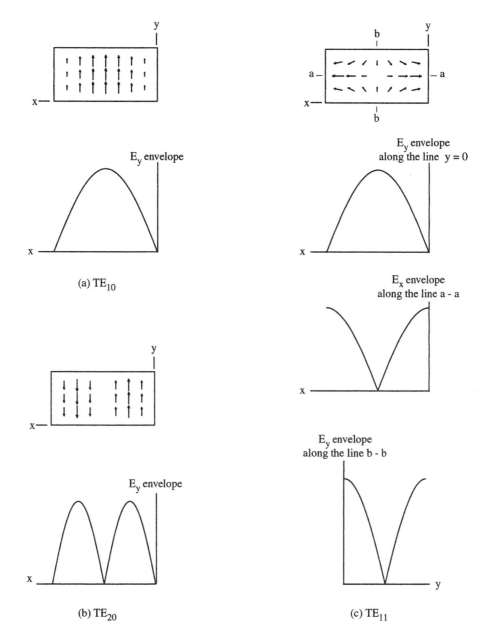

FIGURE 3.40 The mode patterns in one cross section of rectangular waveguide at one instant of time and corresponding envelopes of **E**, for the TE_{10}, TE_{20}, and TE_{11} modes. The envelopes in (a) and (b) are the same for any horizontal line across the waveguide because in the TE_{10} and TE_{20} modes there is no variation with y. In (c), the envelopes are along the lines indicated.

$b = a/2$, where b is the height and a is the width of the waveguide. $b = a/2$ is the condition for which the greatest separation between the TE_{10} and the next modes occurs.

Usually conditions are chosen so that only one mode will propagate in the waveguide, with all the rest of the modes being evanescent. The frequency is therefore adjusted so that it is above the cutoff frequency for the mode with the lowest cutoff frequency (the TE_{10} in Figure 3.42) but below the cutoff frequency of the next modes (the TE_{01} and TE_{20} in Figure 3.42). Then many evanescent modes will exist near the exciting probe and near any discontinuities in the waveguide, but in the

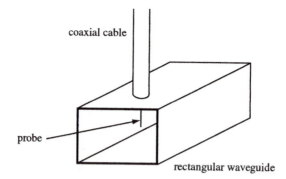

FIGURE 3.41 Diagram of a method of coupling from coaxial cable into rectangular waveguide. The probe excites **E** fields in the waveguide.

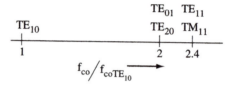

FIGURE 3.42 Cutoff frequencies for various modes normalized to the cutoff frequency of the TE_{10} mode in a rectangular waveguide in which the height is one-half the width.

smooth and regular waveguide, only the propagating mode will exist. This situation is usually desirable because a combination of propagating modes with different amplitudes and different velocities of propagation produce complicated field patterns that are difficult to implement and control.

The cutoff frequency for the TE_{10} mode occurs when $a = \lambda_{co}/2$, where λ_{co} is the free-space wavelength at the cutoff frequency. Because wavelength is inversely proportional to frequency (see Equation 1.25), a smaller waveguide is used at higher frequencies. For example, if $f = 10$ GHz and it is desired that this frequency be halfway between f_{co} for the TE_{10} mode and the next higher mode (see Figure 3.42), then f_{co} for the TE_{10} mode should be 6.67 GHz, for which λ_{co} is given by $\lambda_{co} = 3 \times 10^8/6.67 \times 10^9 = 0.045$ m. Thus the waveguide should be 0.0225 m wide and 0.01125 m high (remember $b = a/2$ in Figure 3.42). For an operating frequency of 20 GHz, the waveguide would be half as large.

3.5.3.3 Waveguide Systems for Exposing Biological Samples

Samples are sometimes placed in various kinds of nonmetallic containers and placed in waveguides to expose them to microwave fields. Considerations of such systems are similar to those discussed in Section 3.5.2 for biological samples placed in TEM systems. The mode patterns in the cross section of waveguide, though, can be considerably different from those in the cross section of TEM systems.

The lossiness of the sample, however, causes the same kind of effects in waveguide exposure systems as those illustrated in Figures 3.35 and 3.36 in connection with TEM exposure systems. In those figures, the magnitude of the voltage is shown as a function of distance in the direction of propagation. In a waveguide exposure system, similar effects apply to the **E** field. It is often difficult to ensure that a biological sample in a waveguide is exposed to uniform fields throughout the sample.

3.6 RESONANT SYSTEMS

Resonance is an effect that is important in the frequency range treated in this chapter. The basic phenomenon of resonance is illustrated by the excitation of the two-dimensional model of a cavity

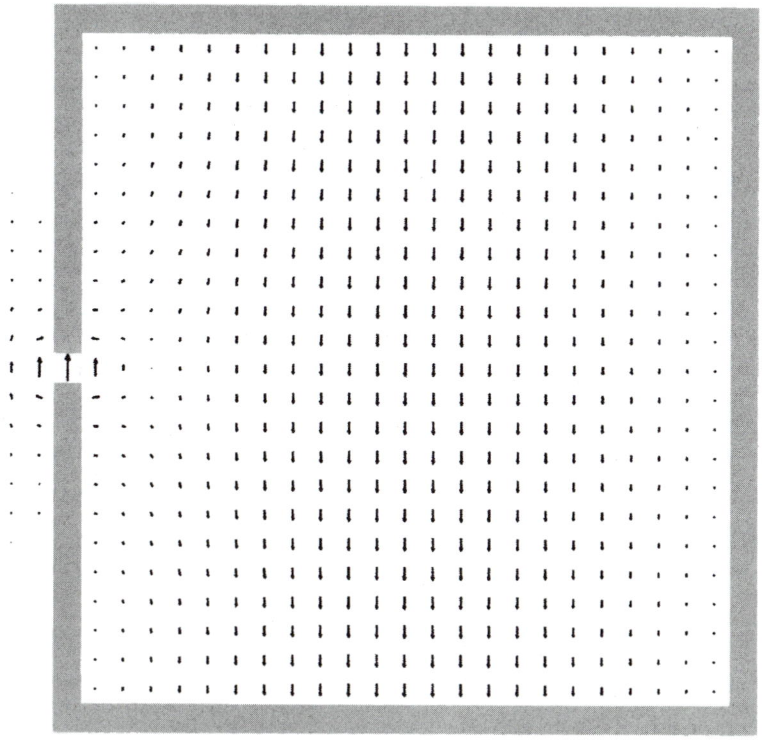

FIGURE 3.43 **E** fields in a two-dimensional model of an air-filled cavity excited by a current source (not shown) connected across the gap in the left cavity wall with a frequency of 670.2484 MHz. The inside dimensions of the cavity walls are 23 cm × 23 cm.

shown in Figure 3.43. A cavity is a hollow enclosure in which EM fields can be excited. Commonly used cavities consist of a section of waveguide, either rectangular or cylindrical, with conducting walls added at each end. EM fields are excited inside the cavity by a probe or loop or some other connection to a source. In the 2D model of Figure 3.43, a current source is connected across the hole in the left wall of the cavity.

The strength of the **E** and **H** fields excited in the cavity is a strong function of the frequency of the source and the size and shape of the cavity. Figure 3.43 shows the **E** fields at one instant of time at the lowest frequency for which the **E** fields are strongly excited (keeping the current source magnitude constant). Figure 3.44 shows an expanded view of the fields inside the cavity. Figure 3.45 shows the response of the cavity as a function of the frequency of the current source when the inside dimensions of the cavity are 23 cm × 23 cm. For the purposes of this illustration, the response of the cavity is defined as the sum of the squares of all the **E** fields inside the cavity, which is proportional to the energy stored in the **E** fields inside the cavity for a fixed source strength. A strong resonance occurs at a frequency of 670.2484 MHz. That is, the response is much stronger at that frequency than at other adjacent frequencies.

Figure 3.46 shows the effects of adding some slightly lossy material to the cavity. The loss in the cavity makes the response curve wider and lower. The relative width of the response curve is called the *bandwidth*. The lossy curve has a wider bandwidth than the lossless curve. When the bandwidth is narrow, the Q of the cavity (Q stands for quality factor) is higher than when the bandwidth is wider. Thus the lossy cavity has a lower Q and a wider bandwidth than the lossless cavity.

Resonance occurs near frequencies for which multiples of half wavelengths fit across the cavity from left to right or from top to bottom. The lowest resonant frequency occurs near the

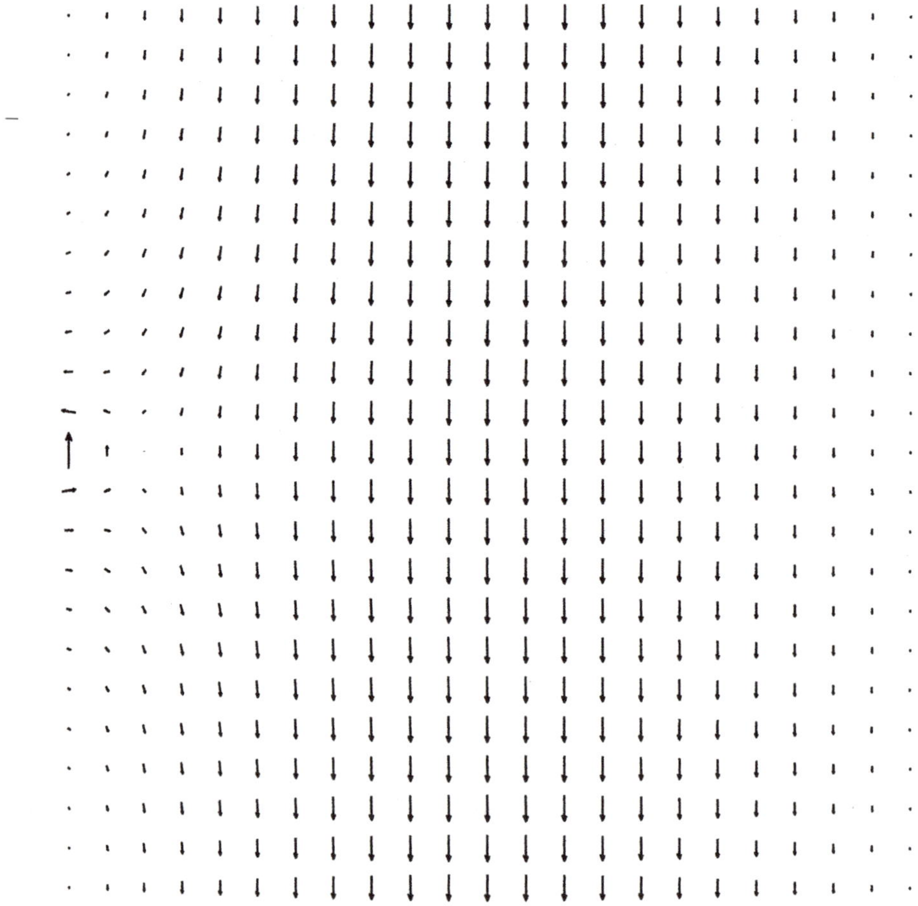

FIGURE 3.44   An expanded view of the **E** fields inside the cavity of Figure 3.43.

frequency at which one half-wavelength occurs from left to right and zero half-wavelengths from top to bottom (i.e., the field does not change from top to bottom). The frequency for which one half-wavelength exactly fits across the cavity is found from Equation 1.25. For $\lambda/2 = 23$ cm, $\lambda = 46$ cm, and $f = c/\lambda = 3 \times 10^8/46 \times 10^{-2} = 652.1739$ MHz. When one half-wavelength fits exactly across the cavity, a null occurs at the left wall and at the right wall, with an envelope like that shown in Figure 3.40(a). However, according to the finite-difference, frequency-domain numerical calculations for the 2D model shown in Figure 3.43, the resonant frequency is 670.2484 MHz, which is about 3% higher than 652.1739 MHz. The reason the resonant frequency is slightly higher than 652.1739 MHz is that the hole in the wall perturbs the pattern slightly, causing a null just to the right of the hole, as shown in Figure 3.44.

Figure 3.47 shows the **E**-field pattern for a higher-order mode at a resonant frequency of 1315.9489 MHz. This pattern shows variation in the fields both from left to right and from top to bottom. Many other resonant frequencies exist for this 2D model with multiple variations in both directions, across and up and down. In actual 3D cavities, multiple resonant frequencies occur with multiple variations in all three directions across the cavity. Similar effects occur in cylindrical cavities, and cavities of other shapes.

The simple 2D model described above illustrates the general characteristics of resonance. EM fields are strongly excited in cavities at very specific frequencies. At other frequencies, the EM fields inside the cavity are only very weakly excited. Cavities are used in many applications where

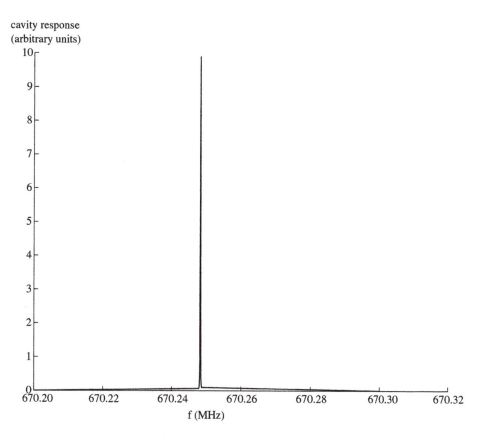

FIGURE 3.45   Cavity response as a function of excitation frequency for the cavity of Figure 3.43. Cavity response is the sum of the squares of all the **E** fields inside the cavity, which is proportional to the energy stored in the **E** fields. A strong resonance occurs at 670.2484 MHz.

frequency discrimination is required, such as in tuners for selecting a signal of a specific frequency out of multiple signals of various frequencies, and in filters that reject signals as a function of frequency.

Biological samples are also sometimes placed in cavities to expose them to EM fields. As illustrated by the example above, however, the loss in the samples will considerably lower the Q of the cavity, lower the fields inside the cavity, and increase the bandwidth. Furthermore, because the **E** and **H** fields in the cavity are generally not very uniform, care must be taken in determining the dosimetry of the EM fields in the sample.

Figure 3.48 shows the cavity response when a biological sample having a conductivity of 0.6 S/m and a relative permittivity of 100 is placed in the center of the cavity. Note from the figure caption that the cavity response in Figure 3.48 is 1 million times weaker than that shown in Figure 3.45 for the empty cavity. The presence of the sample has changed the resonant frequency markedly, as well as lowered the Q and increased the bandwidth. Figure 3.49 shows the **E** fields inside the cavity at the resonant frequency of 644.937 MHz. The pattern shows a perturbation of the pattern of the empty cavity, with the **E** fields inside the sample much weaker than those outside, which would be expected because the conductivity and relative permittivity of the sample are both relatively high. Also, the phase of the **E** fields in Figure 3.49 relative to the current source is about 90° offset from the phase of the **E** fields in the empty cavity relative to the current source. This phase difference is caused by the high relative permittivity of the sample in the cavity. An understanding of resonance effects is obviously important in designing experiments and interpreting results.

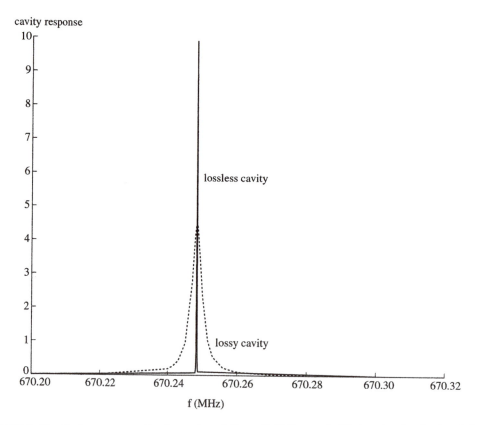

FIGURE 3.46 Cavity responses for the cavity of Figure 3.43 for an air-filled cavity (lossless) and for a cavity filled with a material having a conductivity of 2×10^{-7} S/m (lossy). The response for the lossy cavity has been multiplied by 100 to make the graph visible on the same set of axes as that of the lossless cavity.

3.7 RADIATION EFFECTS

As explained in Section 1.14, when the wavelength is on the order of the size of the system, energy can be efficiently beamed through the air, as well as transmitted through coaxial cables and waveguides. A typical system for transmitting EM signals through the air consists of a source, such as a radio transmitter or microwave generator, a transmission line or waveguide, and an antenna. The source produces EM fields that propagate along the transmission line or waveguide to the antenna, which launches the propagating wave into space, where it propagates similarly to how the waves described in the first part of this chapter propagate. Such antennas are called *transmitting antennas*. Antennas are also used to receive EM radiation, which is then propagated along a transmission line to a receiver. These antennas are called *receiving antennas*. An antenna can usually be used as either a transmitting antenna or a receiving antenna. This section describes some of the general properties and characteristics of antennas.

Antennas are classified into several groups: wire antennas, aperture antennas, array antennas, reflector antennas, and lens antennas. Wire antennas are various combinations of wires or rods. Some commonly used ones are shown in the upper portion of Figure 3.50. A dipole antenna consists of two segments of rod or wire, with a transmission line connected between them. The tip-to-tip length of a dipole antenna is typically one-half of a wavelength. A folded dipole, as the name indicates, is a dipole with an additional connection between the ends. Loop antennas may be circular, square, or other shapes.

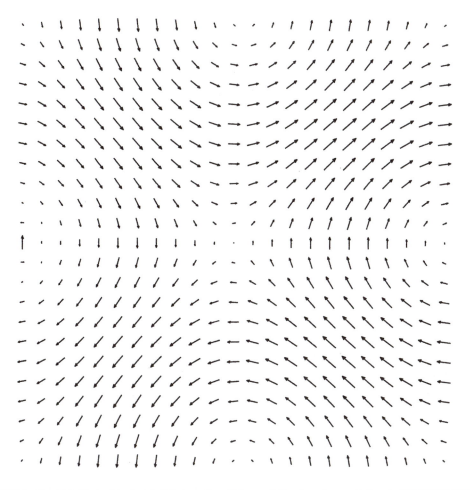

FIGURE 3.47   **E** fields inside the air-filled cavity of Figure 3.43 when the excitation is 1315.9489 MHz.

Aperture antennas are openings through which EM waves are launched into space, such as horns, like the pyramidal horn shown in the lower part of Figure 3.50, open-ended waveguides, slots in waveguides, or other kinds of apertures. Array antennas are arrays of various kinds of antennas, such as a series of dipole antennas. TV-receiving antennas are usually array antennas, with one of the rods being the active, or driven element, and the other rods serving as directors or reflectors of EM radiation. A series of slots in a waveguide is another kind of array antenna.

A typical reflector antenna is the parabolic microwave dish commonly used to receive TV signals from satellites. The parabolic reflector concentrates the microwave energy at its focal point. Lens antennas are used to form EM radiation into beams for transmission into space or to receive and concentrate EM radiation. Because lens antennas must be large compared with a wavelength if they are to be effective, they are used primarily at higher frequencies, where wavelengths are smaller.

Directional antennas transmit or receive radiation more effectively in some directions than others. *Isotropic antennas* transmit or receive radiation equally in all directions. Only ideal antennas (e.g., a point source), not physically realizable antennas, are truly isotropic. *Radiation patterns* are used to describe the characteristics of antenna radiation or reception. Radiation patterns can be either *field patterns* or *power patterns*. Field patterns show either the **E** field or the **H** field as a function of position, and power patterns show the power as a function of position. Fields near the

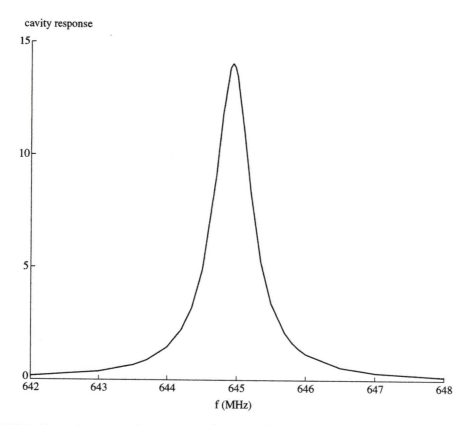

FIGURE 3.48 Cavity response for the cavity of Figure 3.43 in which a biological sample with a conductivity of 0.6 S/m and a relative permittivity of 100 has been placed. This response is about a million times weaker than that of Figure 3.45 (the relative scale here differs from the one in Figure 3.45 by a factor of a million).

antenna are called *near fields*, and fields farther away from the antenna are called *far fields*. The distance from the center of the antenna to where the far fields begin is given by

$$R = \frac{2D^2}{\lambda}, \tag{3.14}$$

where D is the largest dimension of the antenna and λ is the wavelength. The near fields vary more rapidly with space than the far fields. **E** and **H** are not necessarily perpendicular in the near fields, and the near fields are not so much like propagating waves. In the far fields, **E** and **H** are perpendicular, and the fields have the characteristics of propagating waves.

Figure 3.51 shows the far-field **E**-field pattern for a thin half-wavelength dipole. The plot is called a polar plot. In a polar plot, each point in the plane is located by two coordinates, the distance out from the origin (center) and the angle from a vertical line. In the radiation pattern, the angle of each point on the curve is the angle at which the magnitude of the **E** field is calculated, and the distance out from the origin represents the relative magnitude of the **E** field at that given angle. The magnitudes of the **E** field are all calculated at a given far distance from the antenna, and that distance does not show up on the plot. In the far fields, the angular dependence of **E** does not depend on the distance away from the antenna.

In any plane containing the antenna of Figure 3.51, the radiation pattern is the same. Thus, looking at the end of the antenna, the radiation pattern would be a circle centered about the antenna. In a 3D representation, the radiation pattern would appear as a doughnut around the antenna.

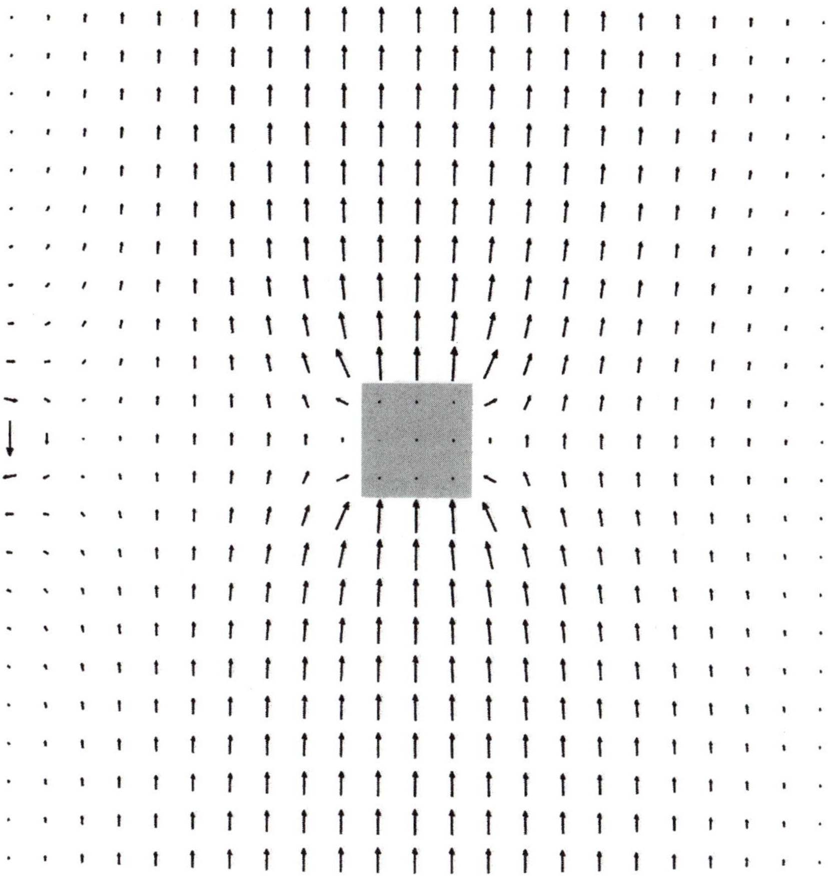

FIGURE 3.49 E fields in the cavity of Figure 3.48 at the resonant frequency of 644.937 MHz.

As shown by Figure 3.51, the maximum radiation occurs broadside to the antenna, that is, at 90° to the antenna. Furthermore, the antenna does not radiate off its ends, as indicated by the nulls in the pattern at 0° and 180°. This is a general characteristic of wire antennas; they do not radiate off their ends. As another example of this characteristic, Figure 3.52 shows the radiation pattern for a dipole antenna that is 1.25 wavelengths long. The pattern shows that no radiation occurs off the end. The pattern also shows an additional effect not seen in Figure 3.51: the presence of *major lobes* and *minor lobes*, or *side lobes*. In some applications, radiation in one direction only is desirable. For example, in transmitting from a fixed radio transmitter to a fixed radio receiver, radiation in other directions is essentially wasted. In these cases, the antenna should be very directional, having one large, narrow lobe and no side lobes. This ideal situation is not usually attainable, but some antennas come close to it.

In other applications, radiation in all directions is desirable. For example, in transmitting from one transmitter to stations in many different locations, an isotropic radiator is desirable. As mentioned above, an isotropic radiator is not physically realizable, but again, some antennas come close to being isotropic.

Bioelectromagnetic research uses antennas of both kinds. In some, a directional antenna is used to expose one animal or one sample. In other applications, antennas with less directionality are used to expose many animals. A basic understanding of the characteristics of antennas is important in designing and interpreting experiments in which antennas are used to expose biological specimens, especially in ensuring satisfactory dosimetry.

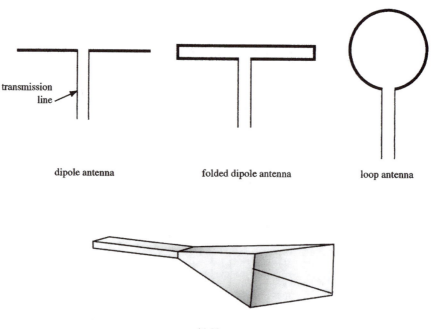

FIGURE 3.50 Examples of antennas. The top three are called wire antennas, and the pyramidal horn is an example of an aperture antenna.

3.8 DIFFRACTION

The simple model of a planewave showed that the planewave will propagate along a straight path perpendicular to its wavefront as it travels through a uniform medium (such as a vacuum or a uniform dielectric) until it hits a reflecting surface or is bent at a refracting interface. This straight-line travel strictly holds, however, only for a planewave, which, according to the definition (see Section 3.2.2), has an infinitely wide wavefront. If the wavefront extent is limited—for example by passing the planewave through a small slit or hole in an absorbing screen—the wave will start spreading outward after it passes through the aperture and will no longer be a planewave. This digression from straight-line travel (other than that caused by reflection or refraction) is termed *diffraction*.

3.8.1 DIFFRACTION FROM APERTURES

The extent of the spreading after passing through an aperture is inversely proportional to the size of the opening expressed in units of wavelength. Therefore, diffraction is not noticeable if the hole or transmitting aperture is many wavelengths wide. Diffraction becomes important only when the aperture is on the order of a few wavelengths or smaller. For the waves discussed in this chapter, the wavelengths range from about a millimeter to several meters, and typical openings may be comparable in size to these wavelengths. In this case, it is necessary to consider diffraction. Optical waves, on the other hand, as discussed in Chapter 4, possess wavelengths that are less than a micrometer, so diffraction occurs only for very small apertures. Diffraction also takes place when waves pass around an edge, wall, or some other single-sided boundary.

As an example of the effects of diffraction, consider the case of a planewave passing through a 2D slit in an otherwise absorbing screen, as shown in Figure 3.53. The slit in this figure is ten wavelengths wide. The effect of the slit on the planewave can be thought of in this way: Each point in the aperture of the slit acts like a point source producing a "wavelet." The transmitted beam is a combination of all those wavelets. This is an expresssion of Huygen's Principle.

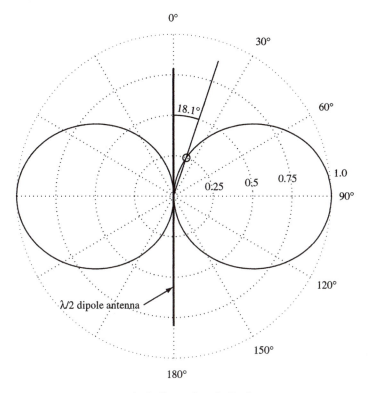

FIGURE 3.51 E-field radiation pattern of a half-wavelength dipole antenna.

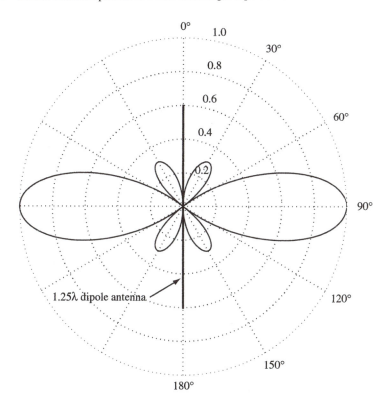

FIGURE 3.52 E-field radiation pattern of a 1.25-wavelength dipole antenna.

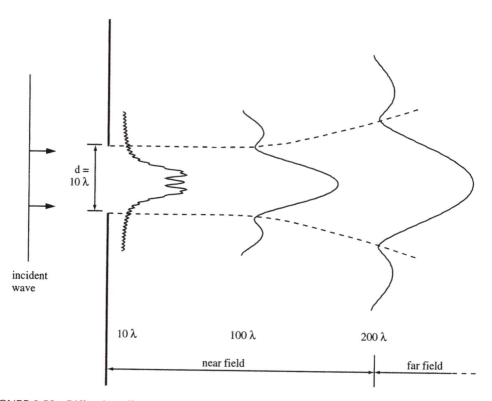

FIGURE 3.53 Diffraction effects on a beam passing through a slit aperture that is ten wavelengths (10 λ) wide. The profiles of the magnitude of **E** are plotted at distances of 10, 100, and 200 wavelengths from the slit. The **E**-field profiles show that the beam pattern is irregular in the near field but becomes smoother in the far field. The horizontal and vertical scales are not equal in this figure.

The transmitted beam's behavior can be divided into two regions. Just after passing through the aperture, the wave has not yet spread out appreciably, and the shadow of the slit still determines the approximate width of the beam. This region close to the slit is called the near field, or Fresnel region, as discussed earlier. One characteristic of this area is the irregular nulls and peaks in the magnitude of the **E** field (and associated **B** field, not shown). These spatial irregularities are caused by constructive and destructive interference among the wavelets propagating from all points in the aperture.

The behavior of the beam changes gradually as it travels away from the aperture going from the near field into the far field. The transition between these two regions is not abrupt, so the definition of this transition distance (already introduced in Equation 3.14) is somewhat arbitrary; it does provide, however, a measure of the extent of the irregular, laterally confined near field.

The first change that is noticeable during the transition into the far field is that the beam field pattern becomes much more regular. The center portion of the beam (the main lobe) takes on a smooth, peaked shape, dropping to a null on both sides before rising again in repetitive side peaks (the side lobes) of rapidly diminishing size. The second change is that the edges of the beam—defined here by the first nulls on both sides of the main lobe as indicated by the dashed line—begin to spread laterally in a fashion that is linearly proportional to the distance from the aperture.

These characteristics (the transition distance and the degree of the linear spreading) are determined by the size of the opening measured in units of wavelength. Figure 3.54 shows diffraction from an aperture that is half the width of that for the previous figure—five wavelengths in this case. Note that the near field still shows irregularities, but over a shorter extent than for the larger slit opening (as predicted by Equation 3.14 using D = d). Also note that the spreading angle in the

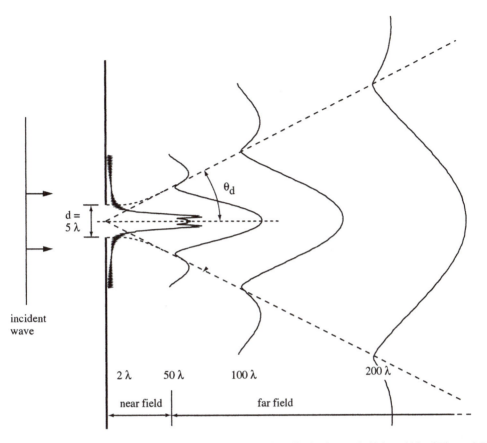

FIGURE 3.54 Diffraction effects on a beam passing through a slit that is one-half the width of Figure 3.53. The extent of the near field is smaller, but the angle of divergence of the **E**-field profile is larger than before.

far field is almost double that of the previous case. This angle, called the half angle of divergence, θ_d, is given for the 2D geometry shown in Figure 3.54 by

$$\sin(\theta_d) = \frac{\lambda}{d}, \tag{3.15}$$

where λ is the wavelength in the medium where the beam is propagating. It is important to note that the angle of spreading is inversely proportional to size of the opening given as a ratio to the wavelength. Thus, the smaller the opening or the longer the wavelength, the larger the spreading. For 3D diffraction (for example from a circular pinhole), the divergence angle and far-field beam pattern are not exactly the same as that produced by a slit, but they show similar qualitative behavior.

The inverse relationship between divergence angle and opening size holds for other situations as well, such as the beam propagating from the output aperture of a radiofrequency power applicator designed for hyperthermia treatment of cancer. At a frequency low enough to penetrate deeply into the body to reach deep tumors, say 100 MHz, the wavelength in muscle is about 30 cm. The aperture of a typical applicator will be on the order of this size, and Equation 3.15 shows that the propagating beam will spread out considerably in the far field, making localized energy deposition impossible at deep locations. Making the aperture smaller results in less radiation efficiency and in even more spreading in the far field, eventually approaching a uniform radiation pattern for a very small aperture like a point source. However, making the aperture smaller does confine the beam to a smaller dimension in the near field (though it is somewhat irregular). These applicators

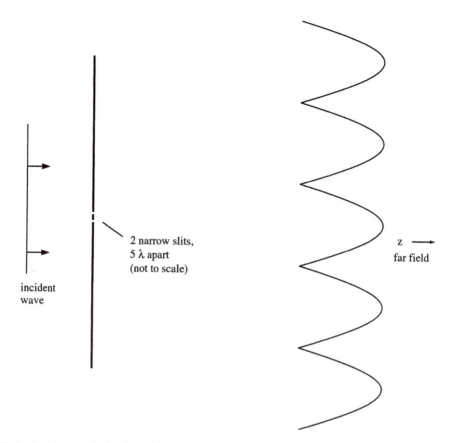

incident
wave

2 narrow slits,
5 λ apart
(not to scale)

z ⟶
far field

FIGURE 3.55 The magnitude of the **E** field in the far field after passing through two narrow slits. Constructive and destructive interference between the waves coming from each slit is responsible for the peaks and valleys.

are better suited to depositing localized electromagnetic heating in superficial tissues than in deep regions. This limitation is discussed more extensively in Section 6.3.1.3.

3.8.2 DIFFRACTION FROM PERIODIC STRUCTURES

An interesting wave interference effect takes place when there is an *array* of uniformly spaced apertures. This phenomenon is shown progressively in Figures 3.55–3.57. In Figure 3.55, the far-field pattern at an observation plane is shown for the radiation from two very narrow slits. (If there were just one narrow slit, the far-field pattern would be very wide with nearly uniform illumination at the observation plane. We have chosen narrow slits in this example, and the previous section has shown that the divergence angle is very large if the slit is narrow compared with the wavelength.) When two slits are present, there are some places on the observation plane where the two fields from the slits add in phase and the resulting **E** field is reinforced, and there are some places in between where the fields add out of phase (subtract really) and are cancelled. The resulting pattern shows broad peaks with nulls in between.

When the number of slits is increased to four with the same center-to-center spacing, as in Figure 3.56, the constructive and destructive interference becomes more pronounced, causing the peaks to become narrower. Each peak is centered at the same position as before because, as will be discussed shortly, the angles to the various peaks are set by the slit spacing in terms of wavelength, which has not changed. When the number of slits increases to 50, the peaks become very pronounced, as shown in Figure 3.57. Employing even more slits makes the peaks extremely narrow.

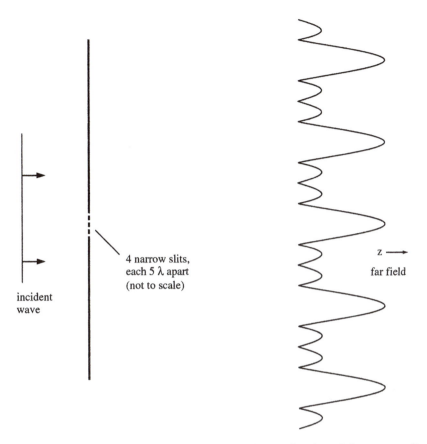

FIGURE 3.56   The magnitude of the **E** field in the far field after passing through four narrow slits with the same spacing as in Figure 3.55. The peaks are narrower, but they are located at the same angles.

The angle of propagation of the peaks is an inverse function of the slit spacing (in units of wavelength). The derivation of this relationship is based on the following principle: The angles of maximum constructive interference (thus the angle of the peaks) are those angles where the paths taken by the waves from each neighboring slit differ by an integral number of wavelengths. The waves, therefore, add in phase when they reach the observation plane. This situation is indicated in Figure 3.58 for two neighboring slits. When the path length difference, Δp, is equal to an integral number of wavelengths, $n\lambda$, trigonometry applied to the triangle gives the angle θ_n of the nth peak with respect to the horizontal axis as

$$\sin \theta_n = \frac{n\lambda}{l} \qquad n = 0, \pm 1, \pm 2K \quad , \tag{3.16}$$

where l is the spacing between the slits.

One of the most practical uses of this effect is the application of diffraction gratings in measuring the wavelength spectrum of an electromagnetic signal, most often in optics. In this case, the array of diffracting elements is usually composed of a grating of narrowly spaced grooves on a surface. When the beam to be analyzed is reflected from the grating, peaks corresponding to the various wavelength components in the beam are displayed on the detection plane at unique angles related to their wavelength by Equation 3.16. There are several spectroscopic uses of light in measuring the chemical or disease state of tissues (many *in vivo*), as discussed in the next chapter, which employ diffraction gratings for the analysis of the optical spectrum reflected or transmitted by the tissues.

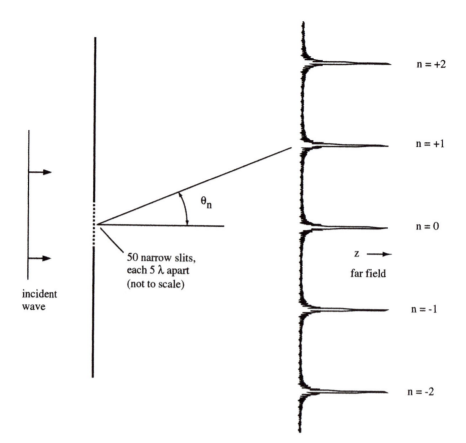

FIGURE 3.57 The magnitude of the **E** field in the far field after passing through 50 narrow slits with the same spacing as in Figure 3.55. The peaks become much narrower as interference from the multiple apertures sharpens the angular response. The peaks are labeled with an index n representing their spacing away from the central (n = 0) peak.

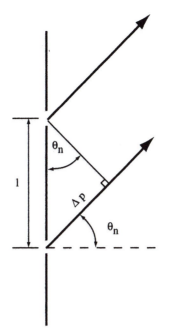

FIGURE 3.58 A simple picture of two neighboring slits, which yields the angles θ_n of maximum constructive interference (i.e., the angles to the peaks). Maximum constructive interference takes place when the path length difference between the two rays, Δp, is an integral number of wavelengths.

4 EM Behavior When the Wavelength is Much Smaller Than the Object

4.1 INTRODUCTION

This chapter discusses the case when the wavelength of the electromagnetic radiation is much smaller than the size of typical objects. Most of the structures encountered in devices such as radiators or detectors lie in the broad range from perhaps a millimeter up to a meter in size. Thus, this chapter concerns waves whose frequencies are high enough that the wavelengths are a millimeter or less. Since f = c/λ (see Section 1.13), the frequency will be in the range of $3 \times 10^8 / 1 \times 10^{-3}$ = 3×10^{11} = 300 GHz and higher. At the lower end of this frequency range are the millimeter waves, so named because their wavelengths are a fraction of a millimeter up to a few millimeters (see Figure 1.23 for a graph of the various electromagnetic regions). At somewhat higher frequencies are the far infrared waves, then the near infrared waves whose wavelengths are on the order of micrometers, named according to their relative closeness to visible light wavelengths. Higher in frequency (shorter in wavelength) is the very important visible wavelength range (between 400 nm and 700 nm), where many significant discoveries and devices such as lasers have been made, undoubtedly due to the significance of light in human vision. Ultraviolet (UV) waves are at slightly higher frequencies. At much higher frequencies are the soft, then hard, x-rays.

All of these waves share some common characteristics, but since the frequency range covered is so broad, there are distinct differences as well. For example, the millimeter waves are often considered to be at the high end of microwaves (Chapter 3) because they use generators, detectors, and waveguides that are often specialized versions of the corresponding microwave devices. On the other end of the range, x-rays possess such high frequencies and short wavelengths (thus their extensive use for medical imaging) that they are not appreciably refracted or slowed down by materials containing dipoles, just absorbed and scattered by atoms, so they behave much differently than lower-frequency electromagnetic waves.

In between these extremes are the *optical* waves, which by most definitions encompass the infrared, visible, and ultraviolet regions. These waves are the main focus of this chapter. They share many common features and, as mentioned, play an important role in human life. Since their wavelengths (approximately one-tenth to several micrometers) are much smaller than the typical object, it is often convenient to describe them in two ways that are different from those used in the previous chapters. The first difference is that diffraction is often unnoticeable for these waves (unless purposely caused by specialized gratings or other very small structures). This is because, as covered in Section 3.8, the degree of diffraction is proportional to the ratio of wavelength to object size. Since the wavelength is short compared with most objects (for example a mirror), diffraction is small and does not play a role in the behavior of the propagating wave. The waves can then be conveniently described by straight-line *ray* propagation, and *ray tracing* makes optical propagation much easier to visualize and determine. This is the domain of *geometrical optics*, where the rays follow geometrical rules. Ray tracing is used extensively in the first half of this chapter.

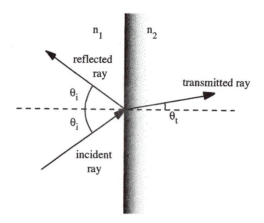

FIGURE 4.1   The refraction (bending) of a ray transmitted through an interface between two dielectrics with refractive indices n_1 and n_2, respectively. In this example, $n_2 > n_1$.

The second difference is that instead of using the permittivity coefficient ε to describe the effect of a material on the propagation of an optical wave, the square root of the relative permittivity ε_r is used. This term is defined as the *index of refraction* n:

$$n = \sqrt{\varepsilon_r}. \tag{4.1}$$

The usefulness of this definition stems from the fact that refraction, as given by Snell's law (Equation 3.5), plays an important role in optics, where lenses are used to focus or change the wavefront curvature of the waves. Snell's law can be conveniently restated in terms of the index of refraction n, or alternatively, the phase velocity v_p. In Figure 4.1, let the wave incident on an interface between two different dielectric materials be represented by its ray at an angle of incidence θ_i (by convention measured with respect to a line perpendicular to the interface). Let the relative permittivity of material 1 be ε_{r1} and the relative permittivity of material 2 be ε_{r2}. After passing through the interface, the angle of transmission is θ_t. Since $\varepsilon_{r1} = \varepsilon_1/\varepsilon_0$ and $\varepsilon_{r2} = \varepsilon_2/\varepsilon_0$ (see Section 1.6), the relationship between the two angles (Equation 3.5) can be formulated in terms of relative permittivity as

$$\sqrt{\varepsilon_{r1}}\,\sin\theta_i = \sqrt{\varepsilon_{r2}}\,\sin\theta_t. \tag{4.2}$$

Then, using the definition of index of refraction Equation 4.1, Snell's law becomes simply

$$n_1 \sin\theta_i = n_2 \sin\theta_t. \tag{4.3}$$

This is the form of the equation usually seen in optical analyses.

Also note that, using Equation 3.4, the phase velocity of the wave in each medium is given by

$$v_{p1} = c/n_1 \qquad \text{and} \qquad v_{p2} = c/n_2. \tag{4.4}$$

Thus the index of refraction is a measure of how much slower a wave is in a medium compared with free space. It follows that Equation 4.3 can equivalently be written as

$$v_{p2} \sin\theta_i = v_{p1} \sin\theta_t. \tag{4.5}$$

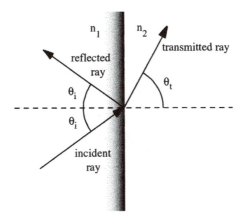

FIGURE 4.2 The refraction (bending) of a ray transmitted through an interface between two dielectrics with refractive indices n_1 and n_2, respectively. In this example, $n_1 > n_2$.

All values of refractive index must be greater than 1, since the law of special relativity states that no energy wave can travel at speeds greater than c, the speed of light in free space (vacuum). Generally, the denser the medium, the higher the index of refraction and the slower the wave speed. Typical values of n are 1.33 for water, approximately 1.5 for glass (depending on the type of glass and the wavelength of the light), and approximately 1.4–1.6 for various transparent plastics. For tissues that have high water content, n is a little higher than 1.33, depending on the density of the proteins, fibers, and other constituents of the tissue. When a substance is lossy, its refractive index becomes a complex number.

4.2   RAY PROPAGATION EFFECTS

As a consequence of the lack of diffraction for most optical waves, as explained in the previous section, the waves will travel in a straight line until reflected (at a mirror, for example) or refracted (by a lens). Due to the smallness of the wavelength, the waves behave like segments of a planewave over any extent of practical interest. Earlier, in Figure 3.3, it was seen that the propagation vector **k** is perpendicular to the wavefront of a propagating planewave. The direction of the propagation vector **k** defines the direction of travel of the wave and is called the *ray* associated with that wave. Thus, when diffraction can be neglected, the ray in a uniform medium travels in a straight line until being redirected.

4.2.1   REFRACTION AT DIELECTRIC INTERFACES

It is useful to use this straight-line ray behavior to describe how optical waves are refracted and focused. For example, Figure 4.1 has already used ray tracing to show how an incident ray is refracted into a different angle after passing through a dielectric interface. For this particular figure, it was assumed that the index of refraction n_1 was smaller than the index n_2, as when going from air ($n_1 = 1$) into water ($n_2 = 1.33$). In this case, the ray is bent more *toward* the normal (perpendicular) direction. As predicted by Equation 4.3, when $n_2 > n_1$, $\sin \theta_i > \sin \theta_t$ and $\theta_i > \theta_t$.

Figure 4.2 shows the opposite case, where n_1 is larger than n_2, as when going from glass ($n_1 = 1.5$) into air ($n_2 = 1$). In this case, the ray bent more *away* from the normal after transmission. It is often useful, when doing ray tracing, to quickly remember which direction a ray will tilt when transmitted in each of these cases. Figure 4.3 gives a very simple, qualitative memory aid for determining the direction of refraction. Think of the ray as being an army tank with two independent treads, one rotating on each side. The tank travels in the direction of the ray. Remember that the speed of the wave (the "tank") is inversely proportional to the index of refraction of the material,

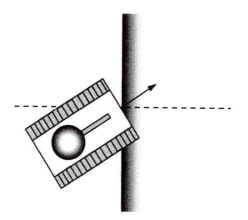

FIGURE 4.3 A simple memory aid to determine which direction a ray will bend when striking a dielectric interface. The army tank represents the incoming wave. One tread will enter region 2 before the other tread and will either be speeded up or slowed down, depending inversely on the relative values of n_1 and n_2. This causes the tank to veer in one direction or the other.

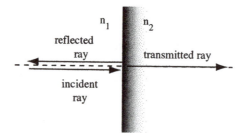

FIGURE 4.4 The situation when a ray strikes the interface at normal incidence (perpendicular to the boundary). Both the transmitted ray and reflected ray are also perpendicular to the boundary, and there is no refraction.

as given by Equation 4.4. Thus, if $n_2 > n_1$ as in Figure 4.1, the speed is slower in medium 2 than in medium 1. Now, as the tank crosses the boundary into medium 2, the right tread will enter first and, therefore, will be slowed down before the left tread is slowed. This will cause the tank to veer more toward the normal, consistent with Snell's law. If $n_1 > n_2$ as in Figure 4.2, medium 2 is faster than medium 1 and the right tread will speed up before the left tread. The tank will veer farther away from normal, again consistent with Snell's law.

Even though this memory aid is very simple, it can be used to obtain Snell's law quantitatively. It also correctly predicts the event when a wave is incident exactly perpendicular to any dielectric interface, as shown in Figure 4.4. In this case, both treads enter at the same time and the tank is not turned either way. In other words, when a wave is incident normally (i.e., perpendicular to an interface), the wave continues on without bending. This is true regardless of the relative magnitudes of the indices of refraction. Of course, Snell's law also predicts this behavior, because when $\theta_i = 0°$, $\sin \theta_i = 0$ and thus $\sin \theta_t = 0$ and $\theta_t = 0°$ independent of the values of either n_1 or n_2. Incidentally, Snell's law also shows that refraction of the incident ray will happen only when n_1 is different from n_2; if the two regions have the same index, there will be no refraction of the ray, as may be intuitively obvious.

Returning to the case when $n_1 > n_2$, Figure 4.2 can be used to predict the onset of total internal reflection (TIR), a phenomenon that has major importance in fiber optics. TIR has been discussed in Section 3.3.2, and here it is reformulated using refractive index terminology. TIR occurs when the incident angle is large enough that the transmitted angle is 90° and essentially the transmitted

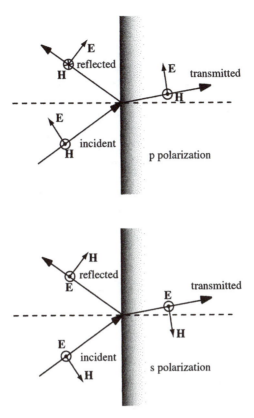

FIGURE 4.5 Definitions of the two independent states of polarization of the incident **E** field. For p polarization, the **E**-field vector lies in the plane of incidence (the plane of the figure). For s polarization, the **E**-field vector is perpendicular to the plane of incidence.

beam disappears. The incident angle at which this happens is called the *critical angle*. It can be found from Equation 4.3 by setting $\theta_t = 90°$ and therefore $\sin \theta_t = 1$. Then

$$\sin \theta_{ic} = \frac{n_2}{n_1}. \qquad (4.6)$$

TIR will take place whenever the incident angle equals the critical angle given by Equation 4.6 or *larger*, including up to an incident angle of 90° (grazing). Over this entire range, there is no transmitted ray into medium 2, only a totally reflected ray in medium 1. Incidentally, because $\sin \theta_{ic}$ has to be smaller than unity for any realizable incident ray, Equation 4.6 shows that TIR will occur only when $n_1 > n_2$, as specified.

4.2.2 OPTICAL POLARIZATION AND REFLECTION FROM DIELECTRIC INTERFACES

The orientation of the incident **E**-field vector defines the *polarization* of the incident wave. As indicated earlier in Figure 3.3, the **E**-field vector will be perpendicular to the direction of propagation of the wave (in most cases of interest in optics) and therefore to the ray. But the orientation of **E** still needs to be specified in the plane perpendicular to the ray. There are two distinct possibilities for the orientation of **E** when dealing with reflection, as shown in Figure 4.5. The plane used for referencing the orientation of **E** is called the *plane of incidence*, and it is defined as the plane that contains both the incident ray and a line drawn perpendicular to the interface (i.e., the dashed line).

In Figure 4.5, the plane of incidence is the plane of the paper. It also contains the reflected ray and the transmitted ray.

When the **E**-field vector is in the plane of incidence, this is *p polarization*. When the **E**-field vector is perpendicular to the plane of incidence (pointing either in or out), this is *s polarization*. Generally, any arbitrary incident polarization can be written as a combination of these two states.

You may have noticed in both Figures 4.1 and 4.2 that, in addition to the transmitted ray, there is also a reflected ray. This is true for all angles of incidence, not just for TIR. As discussed in Section 3.3.2 for microwaves, the angle of reflection equals the angle of incidence to match boundary conditions at all locations along the interface. The amplitude of the reflected wave is found from the *Fresnel* formulae; therefore, reflection from a dielectric interface is called *Fresnel reflection*. The magnitude of the reflection is specified by the amplitude reflection coefficient ρ, which is the ratio of the amplitude of the reflected **E** field to the amplitude of the incident **E** field. ρ depends strongly on the two refractive indices, the angle of incidence, and the polarization of the incident wave.

For p-polarized light, the amplitude reflection coefficient is

$$\rho = \frac{\tan(\theta_i - \theta_t)}{\tan(\theta_i + \theta_t)}, \tag{4.7}$$

where the value of θ_t can be obtained from Snell's law. In the limit of normal incidence (i.e., for $\theta_i = 0°$), Equation 4.7 reduces to

$$\rho = \frac{n_2 - n_1}{n_2 + n_1}. \tag{4.8}$$

For s-polarized light, the amplitude reflection coefficient is

$$\rho = \frac{-\sin(\theta_i - \theta_t)}{\sin(\theta_i + \theta_t)}. \tag{4.9}$$

In the limit of normal incidence ($\theta_i = 0°$), Equation 4.9 reduces to

$$\rho = \frac{n_1 - n_2}{n_1 + n_2}. \tag{4.10}$$

When ρ has a negative value, the amplitude of the reflected wave is 180° out of phase from the incident wave.

These reflection coefficients (ρ) are for the **E** field. To get the *power* reflection coefficient R, or *reflectivity* (the ratio of reflected power density to incident power density), ρ must be squared, since power density is proportional to E^2, as explained in Section 3.4.3. Thus $R = \rho^2$.

As predicted by Equations 4.7 through 4.10, there is some amount of reflection whenever an optical wave passes from one dielectric medium into another. That is why you can see a faint reflection of yourself whenever you look through a glass window. There are actually two separate reflections, one from the front air–glass interface and one from the back glass–air interface. Assuming normal incidence and putting typical values for the indices of air ($n_1 = 1$) and glass ($n_2 = 1.5$) into Equation 4.8 gives $\rho = 0.2$, so $R = \rho^2 = 0.04$. Thus, 4% of the incident power is reflected from the front surface of the glass. Interchanging the roles of n_1 and n_2 changes the sign of ρ. But because $R = \rho^2$, there is no difference in the magnitude of R, so 4% is also reflected from the back surface

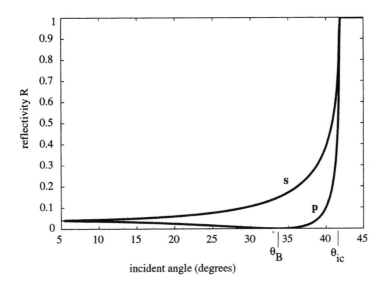

FIGURE 4.6 The variation of the power reflectivity R from a dielectric interface as a function of the angle of incidence. In this example, $n_1 = 1.5$ (glass) and $n_2 = 1$ (air). Note that p-polarized light has zero reflectivity at Brewster's angle (33.7° for this example). Also, note the rise to TIR at the critical angle (41.8° for this example).

and 8% of the power is reflected by both surfaces combined. In some situations, such as with eyeglasses, special antireflection coatings can be put on the glass to reduce this amount to nearly zero.

There are two special cases of reflection that can be determined (with some effort) from Equations 4.7 and 4.9. First, for both polarization states, $\rho \to 1$ when $\sin \theta_i = n_2/n_1$. This, of course, is just a restatement of the condition for TIR discussed earlier. Since $\rho = 1$, it shows that reflection really is *total* (i.e., it is 100% — not merely 99% or 99.99%), as the name "total internal reflection" implies.

The second special case occurs only for p polarization. *Brewster's angle* θ_B is defined as that angle of incidence at which

$$\tan \theta_B = n_2/n_1 . \qquad (4.11)$$

At this special angle of incidence, the magnitude of the reflected wave given by Equation 4.7 goes identically to zero; there is no reflected power. As an example, Figure 4.6 plots the variation of R as a function of the angle of incidence for both polarization states for $n_1 = 1.5$ and $n_2 = 1$. The drop in reflectivity to zero at Brewster's angle can clearly be seen for the p-polarized light, as can the rise to unity at the critical angle for both polarization states for TIR.

4.2.3 RAY TRACING WITH MIRRORS AND LENSES

Optical mirrors are generally made of conductive metal coatings (such as aluminum) on a substrate such as glass. The reflection of optical waves from conductive coatings follows the same boundary conditions as for lower-frequency microwaves (see Section 3.3.1). The reflectivity R depends upon the conductivity of the coating, but it is generally around 90% for aluminum, higher for silver and gold. As before, the angle of reflection equals the angle of incidence. This is known as *specular* reflection. It makes it easy to see the paths of the reflected rays from mirrors. For example, Figure 4.7 shows parallel incident rays reflected from both a flat mirror and a spherical mirror. Since the spherical mirror surface is curved inward (concave), specular reflection causes

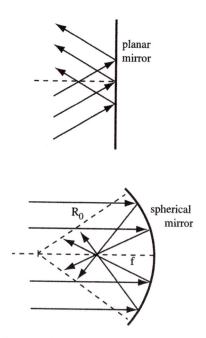

FIGURE 4.7   Reflection of rays from two kinds of mirrors: planar and concave. The concave mirror focuses parallel incoming rays to a distance f halfway between the mirror and its center of curvature.

the parallel rays to focus to a point halfway between the center of curvature and the mirror surface. (This is strictly true only for rays near the axis; for rays farther away from the axis, some spreading of the focus spot, known as *aberration*, occurs.) Thus, for a concave spherical mirror, the focal length f is equal to one-half the radius of curvature R_0, or $f = R_0/2$.

Lenses are most often used to focus or expand light beams. The direction and degree of curvature of the lens surface determines, following Snell's law (Equation 4.3), the amount of focusing of the lens and whether it will converge or diverge an incoming beam. Several varieties of lenses are shown in Figure 4.8. If a lens causes an incoming parallel set of rays (called a *collimated* beam) to converge, it has a positive focal length and is called a *positive* lens. If the lens causes the collimated beam to diverge, it has a negative focal length and is a *negative* lens.

The labeling of lenses usually obeys the following convention: The nature of the curvature of the first surface of the lens viewed from one side (concave, convex, or plano) is given, then the curvature of the other lens surface as viewed from the *other* side is given. Thus a convex-convex lens (sometimes called a double-convex lens) has two surfaces that bulge out at the center, as in the upper left of Figure 4.8. Using Snell's law (or qualitatively, the "tank" memory aid), you can easily trace a ray through a convex-convex lens to see that it will refract a ray originally parallel to the axis to a focal point on the axis on the other side of the lens; therefore it is a positive lens.

Figure 4.8 shows several common lenses, both positive and negative. For thin lenses, it does not matter significantly which orientation a lens takes with respect to the propagation direction of the rays. In other words, if you turn a plano-convex lens around to make it a convex-plano, it will still focus the incoming rays to the same spot. However, aberrations are reduced if the collimated beam strikes the convex surface first, then passes through the planar surface second; i.e., it passes in the direction shown in the upper right of Figure 4.8. This keeps the maximum refraction angle encountered by any ray to a smaller value than if the lens were the other way around.

The focusing power of a lens is determined by both the degree of curvature and the index of refraction of the lens material. Thus a lens with steeper curvature (or two curved surfaces instead of just one) will focus more strongly; this is indicated by a shorter focal length, f. Also, a lens with a higher refractive index will focus more strongly than one with lower index. This is why lightweight

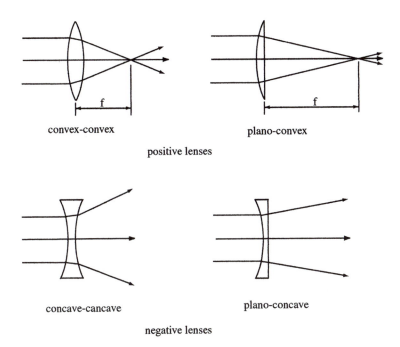

FIGURE 4.8 Examples of both positive and negative focal length lenses; f is the focal length of the lens. The convention for naming the lenses is given in the text.

plastic eyeglass lenses are sometimes made of polycarbonate material; the high refractive index of polycarbonate (n = 1.6) allows the lenses to be curved less (with corresponding lower overall thickness and weight) than with glass or lower index plastics.

A common way to specify the focusing power (or equivalently, the light gathering capability) of a lens is by its f-number, sometimes given as f# or f/. The f-number of a lens is defined by

$$f\# = f/D, \tag{4.12}$$

where f is the focal length of the lens and D is the diameter of the lens or the diameter of a limiting pupil, whichever is smaller. The *smaller* the f-number, the *bigger* the cone of focused rays, or, when used to collect light from a broad-angle source, the *more* light the lens will accept.

4.2.4 IMAGING WITH LENSES

Of course, the major use of lenses in optics is to form images of objects, as in telescopes or cameras. It is beyond the scope of this book to cover imaging in any detail, but Figure 4.9 shows a simple imaging configuration in which the image of an arrow is formed by a positive lens (in this case, a plano-convex lens). There is some magnification M of the image size l_i compared with the original object size l_o; the magnification is defined as $M = l_i / l_o$. For a given imaging setup, the magnification is determined by the ratio of the image distance d_i to the object distance d_o, or $M = d_i / d_o$, as can be seen by using similar triangles in Figure 4.9.

You can quickly get the position of the image by the following simple ray tracing procedure: Trace one ray from some point on the object (say the arrow tip, the ray labeled "a") through the center of the lens; it will not be bent overall (for a thin lens) since it passes directly through the lens center. Then trace another ray from the same point (ray "b") that goes parallel to the axis until it passes through the lens; because it is initially parallel to the axis, the lens will redirect it through the lens focal point, at a distance f from the lens. Where these two rays cross on the other side of

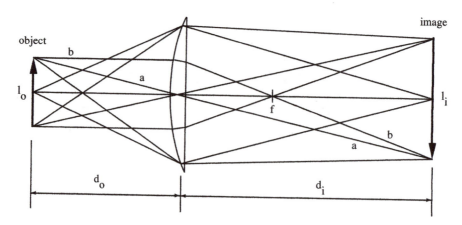

FIGURE 4.9 A simple imaging arrangement using a thin plano-convex lens. The image of the object is magnified by an amount M. The intersection of the rays labeled "a" and "b" determines the location of the image, as explained in the text.

the lens, the image of the chosen object point will be formed. Other rays from the same object point will also meet at this image point (in the absence of aberrations). Then d_i can be measured, and therefore M determined.

The *lens law* can also be used to solve for the image distance d_i. The lens law relates the three distances important in image formation for a thin lens:

$$\frac{1}{d_i} + \frac{1}{d_o} = \frac{1}{f}. \tag{4.13}$$

Specifying two of the three distances will allow you to solve for the third.

4.2.5 GRADED-INDEX LENSES

There is a circumstance in which a ray will *not* follow straight-line propagation, even though diffraction can be neglected. This is the case when the ray is traveling in a medium whose refractive index is not uniform, but rather varies spatially. This type of medium has a graded refractive index, and the ray will follow a curved path whose direction and degree of curvature depend on the index profile.

One of the practical uses of this concept is in the *graded-index lens*, or GRIN lens. Here the focusing power of the lens is not provided by curved faces, but by the graded variation of the lens's refractive index. Usually made from doped glass, the lens has a high index at the center, and the index decreases radially toward the edges. A ray will then take a path similar to that shown in Figure 4.10. The ray will follow the path that gives the shortest propagation time between two points (say A and B in Figure 4.10); this is known as Fermat's principle. Because the velocity of the ray is inversely proportional to the index of refraction, as explained in the introduction, the propagation time is shortened by a path that takes the ray out into the lower-index margins rather than going straight through the high-index center. As seen in the figure, rays coming from a point at one location on one side of the lens will be refocused to a point on the other side of the lens. The GRIN lens thus acts as a true lens and can be used in situations where a regular lens is not suitable.

The GRIN lens is usually much smaller than a regular spherical lens and is often used at the ends of optical fibers (next section) and employed in endoscopes or in other applications where the light from a fiber must be focused, as in fibers for laser light delivery to tissues. GRIN lenses can also be fabricated to have less aberration than regular spherical lenses.

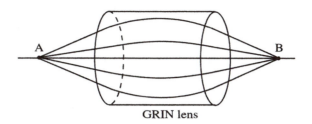

GRIN lens

FIGURE 4.10 A graded-index lens, or GRIN lens, which refracts rays by index variation rather than surface curvature.

optional buffer layer

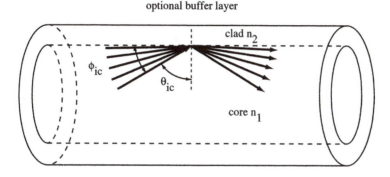

FIGURE 4.11 The structure of a multimode optical fiber. The core refractive index n_1 must be greater than the clad index n_2 to have TIR between the core and the clad. All rays traveling inside at angles that are less than the critical angle ϕ_{ic} with respect to the boundary will be trapped, as shown by the cone of rays.

4.3 TOTAL INTERNAL REFLECTION AND FIBER-OPTIC WAVEGUIDES

One of the most important and practical uses of total internal reflection (TIR) is in optical waveguides. When these waveguides are round glass or plastic fibers, they are known as optical fibers or fiber-optic waveguides. We will use glass fibers as the main example of optical waveguides, although other geometrical forms, such as planar waveguides, are also sometimes seen.

The side view of a round optical fiber is shown in Figure 4.11. The central region of the fiber, known as the *core*, is composed of glass with refractive index n_1. The diameter of the core depends upon whether the fiber is intended to be multimode or single-mode (discussed later); multimode fibers have diameters that generally range from 50 to 200 μm. Formed around the core is a layer of lower refractive index glass, called the *clad*, with refractive index n_2. This forms a step-index fiber. It is essential that $n_1 > n_2$ for TIR to occur. When this is the case, rays inside the core will be trapped by TIR if they strike the core-clad interface at shallow enough angles. From Section 4.2.1, remember that TIR will occur whenever a ray is incident on a dielectric interface with an angle (measured with respect to the perpendicular) that is at or exceeds the critical angle given by Equation 4.6.

It is often convenient in waveguides to define angles with respect to the boundary plane (interface plane), denoted by ϕ, rather than with respect to the perpendicular line, denoted by θ. Thus ϕ and θ are complementary angles and add to 90°. Rewriting the critical angle equation in terms of this angle gives

$$\cos\phi_{ic} = \frac{n_2}{n_1}. \tag{4.14}$$

Then all rays that are propagating inside the core at angles that are at or *less* than ϕ_{ic} with respect to the boundary will be trapped by TIR and will remain inside the core until they reach the end of the fiber and radiate out the end face. This is indicated in Figure 4.11 by a cone of trapped light rays. The attenuation of light by modern glass fibers (due to absorption and scattering) is very low, around 3 dB/km for visible light and less than 0.2 dB/km for certain infrared wavelengths, so very little light is lost. As emphasized in an earlier section, TIR means *total* reflection, so no light is lost by transmission out the sides of the fiber (unless the fiber is tightly bent; then there may be some so-called bending losses).

The need for the clad layer may be puzzling because if the core passes through air (thus $n_2 = 1$), the condition that $n_1 > n_2$ for TIR would surely be met. This is quite true if it could be assured that air would always surround the fiber. But in practical situations, the core will touch other objects, such as metal, plastic, or even fluids. At these locations, n_2 may then be greater than n_1, and TIR would be frustrated and the previously trapped rays would be lost out the side of the fiber. The presence of the clad avoids this possibility by protecting the core-clad interface. How thick should the cladding be? Although the simple ray picture does not predict it, not all the **E** field of the trapped rays is confined to the core. A small portion of the field, called the *evanescent tail*, extends a few hundred nanometers into the clad region. To protect this field from interacting with foreign substances, the cladding layer is made several micrometers thick. The clad must also be transparent. Otherwise it will absorb some of the evanescent tail, taking energy out of the propagating rays and significantly increasing attenuation.

In addition, an optional buffer layer may be placed around the cladding. This coating, which is often a colored organic layer, has no primary optical purpose; it is used to mechanically protect the glass core and clad from scratches and abrasion that would weaken the fiber.

4.3.1 MULTIMODE OPTICAL FIBERS

In a multimode fiber, the rays within the TIR cone in Figure 4.11 comprise various propagating modes of the fiber (similar to the waveguide modes described in Section 3.5.3). Each mode propagates at a unique angle that is slightly different from the neighboring modes. In a typical multimode fiber, however, there are so many modes (thousands) that they appear to be almost continuous in angle.

How many of the possible modes are excited in a given fiber depends on the input conditions. Light is usually coupled into the front face of the fiber from a source such as a laser, a light-emitting diode (LED), or a white-light source like a quartz-halogen incandescent bulb. The beam from a laser is very directional (narrow in angle), so only a few of the allowed fiber modes may be excited at the input. After propagating a distance in the fiber, however, these modes will gradually couple to other angles by scattering and bending of the fiber, and the excited mode structure will start to fill in. When the source is an LED or a bulb, the light emitted from the source is already broad in angle, and usually all the possible modes are excited at the input to the fiber.

The light that radiates from the exit end of the fiber (when the fiber mode structure is full or almost full) comes out as a cone of light that can be related to the cone of modes inside the core. This situation is depicted in Figure 4.12. The cone of angles inside the core is broadened somewhat according to Snell's law of refraction as it exits the flat face of the fiber into the air. The half-angle of the radiated cone in air is given by

$$\sin \phi_r = \sqrt{n_1^2 - n_2^2}. \qquad (4.15)$$

This radiation cone angle can also be put in terms of the numerical aperture NA of the fiber. The numerical aperture is defined as $NA = \sqrt{n_1^2 - n_2^2}$, so Equation 4.15 can also be written as

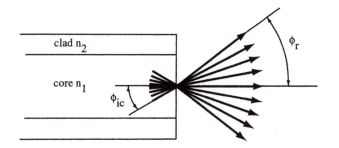

FIGURE 4.12 The exit conditions of rays radiating from the flat end of a multimode fiber. ϕ_r is the half-angle of divergence, assuming all modes (i.e., all allowed propagation angles inside the core) are excited by the source.

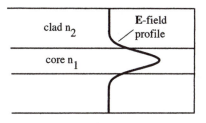

FIGURE 4.13 The E-field pattern for the lowest-order mode (the only allowed mode) of a single-mode fiber. The core diameter is very small (typically about 6–8 µm). The mode shape can be approximated by a Gaussian profile.

$$\sin \phi_r = NA. \qquad (4.16)$$

For example, if $n_1 = 1.55$ and $n_2 = 1.51$, the numerical aperture of the fiber is NA = 0.35 and the half-angle of divergence is 20.5° in air. The full divergence angle is therefore 41°.

4.3.2 SINGLE-MODE OPTICAL FIBERS

The core diameter of a single-mode fiber, about 6–8 µm, is much smaller than that of a multimode fiber. This means only one mode will propagate in the fiber; all others are cut off, analogous to the cutoff condition already seen for microwave waveguides (Section 3.5.3.2). When there is only one mode, the ray picture used for multimode fibers is not adequate and a full wave analysis must be used. The E-field profile for a single-mode fiber is shown in Figure 4.13. There is a central peak in the E-field magnitude, similar to that of the TE_{10} mode of a microwave waveguide (see Figure 3.40). However, in the case of a glass fiber, the E field does not go to zero at the dielectric interface as it must at the metal wall of a microwave waveguide. There is some penetration of the field into the clad region. This is the evanescent tail discussed earlier. Another difference is that the lowest-order mode of the fiber is cylindrically symmetric.

The radiation from the end of a single-mode fiber does not follow the same equation as for multimode fibers because there is no cone of rays in the single-mode fiber. Instead, the mode structure for the single-mode fiber shown in Figure 4.13 closely resembles a Gaussian profile, which will be covered in Section 4.4, that stretches somewhat beyond the core (perhaps 20–50%, depending on the fiber parameters). Thus, the radiation angle is similar to that for a Gaussian beam whose radius is approximately 1.2 to 1.5 times the core radius. The discussion of this radiation angle is deferred until Section 4.4.3, but for typical values, it will be shown that the divergence from a single-mode fiber is less than from multimode fibers.

4.3.3 Applications of Optical Fibers

The largest use of optical fibers today is in telecommunications—most telephone calls and computer hookups are over fibers. Due to speed and distance requirements, almost all of these telecommunication fibers are single-mode.

In biology and medicine, however, most fibers are multimode because they are usually designed to carry light with high collection efficiency. Here fibers find three main applications:

1. Endoscopes are image-transmission devices for peering inside the body. Bundles of thousands of small, closely packed multimode fibers are used to transmit the image. Each fiber transmits the intensity of one small segment (pixel) of the image. Some additional fibers in the bundle are used to carry illuminating light from the outside to the internal location. Since fibers can be bent, the endoscope is often flexible.
2. Fibers are used to deliver laser energy to tissues for laser surgery in dermatology, photodynamic cancer therapy, and other power delivery applications. Again the fibers are flexible for convenient application. Included in this category are fibers for delivery of optical power for ablation of arterial plaque or for other tissue ablation. When the laser is a high-power CO_2 laser (10.6 μm infrared wavelength), the fibers must be fabricated from special infrared-transmitting materials because glass strongly absorbs at this wavelength.
3. Fiber-based sensors for blood gases, blood proteins, and physical parameters such as pressure and temperature are being developed for *in vivo* measurements. The fibers allow direct placement of the sensors in tissues, veins, and arteries.

4.4 PROPAGATION OF LASER BEAMS

As mentioned in the introduction, ray tracing is a very useful tool when diffraction is negligible. But when the beam size is small—as it is when generated from inside the active region of a laser—diffraction must be taken into account and ray tracing is not appropriate. This section discusses the kind of beams that radiate from lasers and how they propagate after leaving the laser.

4.4.1 Linewidths of Laser Beams

One key characteristic that differentiates a laser beam from the beams that come from incandescent bulbs or LEDs is that its wavelength spectrum is much narrower. For optical sources, the wavelength spread is usually called *linewidth*. While a typical LED may have a linewidth that spans 30–40 nm, the spectrum of a laser diode (a semiconductor laser) may span only a fraction of a nm, depending on the number of cavity modes present. Gas lasers (such as the HeNe laser) are even narrower in linewidth. Therefore, the laser beam has a more precisely defined wavelength than the other sources. It is said that the laser has a higher degree of temporal coherence.

Figure 4.14 shows the output spectrum of a typical visible laser diode. In the case shown, the laser has two modes, each at a unique frequency stemming from the resonance of the optical cavity that makes up the laser diode (analogous to the resonant wavelengths of a microwave cavity, discussed in Section 3.6). However, the number and position of the modes of a laser diode often vary in time, especially if the temperature of the diode is not kept constant. This phenomenon is known as *mode hopping*.

4.4.2 The Gaussian Spherical Profile

Another key characteristic of a laser beam is that it is generated by stimulated emission that builds up inside the optical cavity (a multiple-pass cavity known as a Fabry-Perot cavity). Because the

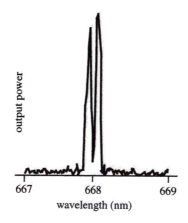

output power

667   668   669

wavelength (nm)

FIGURE 4.14 Example of the output spectrum from a visible laser diode. Two modes are evident here, but some laser diodes have only one (single-mode lasers). The number, strength, and wavelength location of the longitudinal modes vary with temperature and drive current.

beam bounces back and forth many times inside the cavity in the process of building up, it takes on a special profile. Only those beam profiles that reinforce themselves upon multiple bounces, i.e., that keep the same shape after propagating back and forth several times, will survive in the laser's output. One important profile that meets this requirement is the *Gaussian spherical* beam, sometimes simply called a Gaussian beam.

The name "Gaussian" refers to the shape of the beam's amplitude in the transverse direction. A Gaussian shape means that the **E**-field amplitude follows a quadratic exponential profile centered on the beam axis:

$$E = E_0 e^{-[r/w(z)]^2} \tag{4.17}$$

where r is the distance from the axis, E_0 is the magnitude of the **E** field on the axis, and w(z) is a parameter that specifies the radius of the beam at a distance z from a landmark location called the *waist*. At the waist, z = 0, w = w_0, and the beam width here is the smallest it gets (thus the name "waist") until it is refocused by lenses. This shape is shown in Figure 4.15. Since a gaussian amplitude does not have sharp edges, the definition of width is somewhat arbitrary. By convention, the beam radius is defined as the point at which the field amplitude has fallen to 1/e (0.37) of its maximum value at the axis; this occurs at r = w(z). Because power density is proportional to the square of the **E** field, the power density will have fallen to $1/e^2$ (0.14) at this radius.

Note that the *diameter* of the beam is twice the radius, or d = 2w(z). Also note that the Gaussian shape is an ideal because mathematically, the **E**-field amplitude never quite gets to zero even for very large distances away from the axis, yet in practice the amplitude must go to zero at some finite distance. However, the energy carried in the extreme tail of the Gaussian profile is small, so very little is lost if the profile is truncated at a reasonable distance from the axis.

The word "spherical" is used to describe the curvature of the wavefront of the beam, which takes on a spherical shape that changes as the beam propagates. The wavefront curvature is another way of specifying the phase of the **E** field of the beam across any plane perpendicular to the direction of propagation. In Figure 4.15, in general the wavefront is curved away from the waist, but at the waist the wavefront is planar (flat). In fact, the two distinguishing characteristics of the waist are 1) the beam is smallest here and 2) the wavefront is planar here. Where the waist occurs in space depends on what components, such as curved mirrors or lenses, change the wavefront curvature of the Gaussian beam; this is covered in more detail in the next two sections.

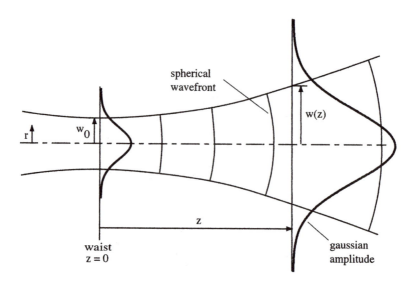

FIGURE 4.15 The propagation of a Gaussian spherical beam away from its waist. The amplitude of the beam at any location z obeys a Gaussian profile with radius w(z). Its wavefront is spherical with varying degrees of curvature. The propagation characteristics are symmetrical in z about the waist; i.e., the converging beam to the left of the waist follows the same shape as the diverging beam to the right.

4.4.3 Propagation Characteristics of a Gaussian Beam

The parameter w(z) defines the radius of a Gaussian beam at any location. As the beam propagates, w(z) will change. It is important to determine how fast w(z) changes because this will determine how fast the beam spreads out (diverges) due to diffraction, or how much the beam will converge when focused. This section looks at diffraction of a beam propagating away from its waist; the next section looks at focusing by a lens.

To examine the propagation of a laser beam, it is first necessary to determine where the waist is located. For almost all lasers, the initial waist is located at or inside the laser cavity, either near the middle or at one of the end mirrors of the cavity. Each laser design will be slightly different. For example, a gas laser will usually have its waist at the output mirror of the laser. A semiconductor laser diode (whose oval output beam is roughly approximated by a Gaussian beam with different waist sizes along each of two axes) will have its waist at the exit facet of the laser.

Once the waist is located, the beam radius can be found by noting that the beam expands monotonically as a function of the distance z away from the waist according to the following formula:

$$w(z) = w_0 \sqrt{1 + \left(\frac{z}{z_R}\right)^2}, \tag{4.18}$$

where z_R is the *Rayleigh range* defined by

$$z_R = \frac{\pi w_0^2}{\lambda}. \tag{4.19}$$

An example of this beam divergence is shown in Figure 4.16. Note from Equation 4.18 that the beam has expanded to just $\sqrt{2}$ of its waist radius when it reaches the Rayleigh range at $z = z_R$. The Rayleigh range is therefore one measure of the extent of the near field of the beam divergence.

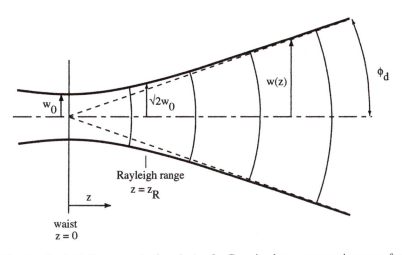

FIGURE 4.16   The far-field divergence half-angle ϕ_d of a Gaussian beam propagating away from its waist. The waist is a landmark feature whose radius w_0 determines how the beam will propagate. The location and radius of the waist are set by optical components forming the beam, such as laser cavities or intervening lenses.

Perhaps the most convenient way to express the spreading of the Gaussian beam is to specify its far-field divergence angle. Note from Figure 4.16 that in the far field (i.e., more than a few Rayleigh ranges away from the waist), the beam edges—as defined by $w(z)$—expand linearly as a function of the distance z from the waist. This means that the beam looks like it is expanding linearly from a point located at the center of the waist. The divergence half-angle ϕ_d, shown in Figure 4.16, can be obtained by letting $z \gg z_R$ in Equation 4.18 and using $\sin \phi_d \approx \tan \phi_d = w(z)/z$. This gives the divergence half-angle as

$$\sin \phi_d = \lambda / \pi w_0 \tag{4.20}$$

Therefore, the smaller the waist size, the larger the divergence angle. This is consistent with the behavior seen earlier in the diffraction of a wave after passing through a small slit (Section 3.8.1).

The curvature of the wavefront also changes as the beam propagates away from the waist. At the waist, the wavefront is planar. As it propagates, it begins to curve slightly outward, then becomes more curved at farther distances. In the far field, the wavefront curvature has a radius that is approximately equal to z, the distance from the waist. Thus the beam approximates a segment of a spherical wave that appears to be emanating from a point centered at the waist. At very far distances, the spherical wavefront begins to look planar.

4.4.4   Focusing a Gaussian Beam with a Lens

When a Gaussian beam passes through a lens, a new waist forms at the focal plane of the lens. This occurs because the curvature of the lens surface modifies the wavefront curvature of the beam by refraction, causing it to converge to a new waist location. (The radius of the beam is not changed immediately when passing through the lens, assuming that the lens diameter is somewhat larger than the beam size so the beam is not clipped.) The diameter of this new waist is then a measure of the focused spot size.

Figure 4.17 shows the focusing configuration. The diameter of the focused spot is twice the new waist radius, or $d_0 = 2w_0$, and is given by

$$d_0 = 1.27 \lambda f / D, \tag{4.21}$$

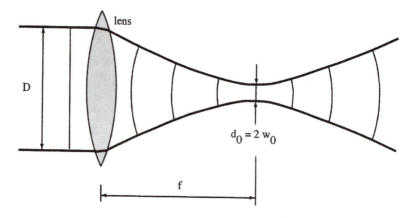

FIGURE 4.17 Focusing of a gaussian beam to a waist by a lens. As opposed to the simple ray picture, where the focused spot can be infinitely small, the actual spot diameter d_0 is finite. It is a function of the beam diameter D, the focal length f, and the wavelength λ.

where f is the focal length of the lens, λ is the wavelength, and D is the diameter of the beam as measured at the lens location. Thus, to make a focused spot smaller, a shorter focal length lens or a larger diameter input beam should be used. However, as mentioned above, the lens diameter must be greater than the beam diameter to avoid clipping, and it is difficult in practice to fabricate a lens whose diameter is much greater than its focal length; otherwise, aberration will be severe. In other words, f/1 is about the smallest f-number possible in a practical lens. Therefore, the smallest value the term f/D in Equation 4.21 can have in practice is approximately unity. In this case, d_0 will then be on the order of the wavelength of the light.

This illustrates a rather universal principal: About the smallest an electromagnetic wave can be focused is on the order of the wavelength of the wave. This sets the ultimate limit on the resolution of conventional optical microscopes and is why short wavelength light is preferred when a small focused size is needed to increase spot density in such applications as CD disks or optical storage. It is also why electrons, with extremely short wavelengths, have such good spatial resolution when used to image objects with the scanning electron microscope.

4.4.5 APPLICATION OF GAUSSIAN BEAM EQUATIONS

The Gaussian beam equations of this section are a very good approximation to the beams from many lasers, such as gas or solid-state (e.g., NdYAG) lasers. For example, the beam exiting a typical HeNe laser has a waist radius of about 1 mm. Since $\lambda = 633$ nm, Equation 4.20 predicts a divergence half-angle of only 0.011° (the full angle would be twice this value). This small amount of divergence is what makes a laser beam look like a "pencil" beam.

The Gaussian equations do not apply quite as well to semiconductor laser diodes because the typical edge-emission laser diode has an emitting junction that is a tiny, flat rectangle rather than a round mirror. But the equations still can be used approximately, with more accuracy in the short-axis dimension of the rectangle than in the long-axis direction. Because the emitting face is rectangular and because divergence is inversely proportional to the emission dimension (as seen in Equation 4.20), there will be more divergence in the laser diode's output beam in the plane perpendicular to the flat junction than in the plane parallel to the junction. As shown in Fig. 4.18, this causes the output beam to become oval, with the long axis of the oval rotated 90° with respect to the long axis of the junction.

As an example, the short-axis dimension of the emitting junction of a typical laser diode may be only about 1.5 μm high. Letting $w_0 = 1$ μm (since the **E** field extends slightly beyond the confines of the junction) and $\lambda = 660$ nm in Equation 4.20 gives a half-angle of divergence in the

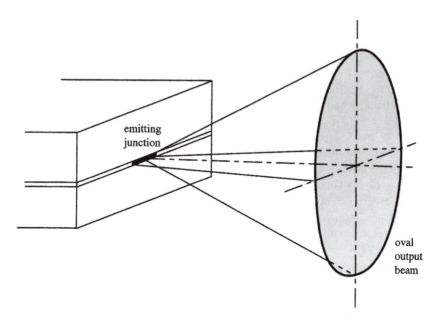

FIGURE 4.18 The output beam of a semiconductor laser diode. Because the emitting junction is rectangular, the divergence angles along the two transverse beam axes are unequal, with the divergence in the plane perpendicular to the junction's small dimension being larger than along the other axis. This leads to an oval output beam unless corrected by special optical components.

plane perpendicular to the junction of 12.1° for a full angle of 24.2°. The long-axis dimension of the junction may be 10 μm wide. Assuming a Gaussian profile along this dimension, Equation 4.20 predicts that the divergence half-angle in the plane parallel to the junction would be 2.4° for a full angle of 4.8°. Actually, because the E-field profile in the long-axis direction is not really Gaussian but is composed of higher-order transverse modes that are flatter in profile, the true divergence angle in this plane is somewhat larger than predicted by Gaussian theory. The equations match closer along the small-axis direction than in the long-axis direction.

The divergence angles from an unfocused laser diode are rather large, as calculated above. To make the beam more directed, a short focal-length lens is often placed close to the junction to collimate the beam. The new divergence angles are based upon the larger waist sizes at the lens, and divergence can therefore be much reduced.

Also, as mentioned in Section 4.3.2, the beam radiating from the face of a single-mode fiber can be approximated quite closely by a Gaussian beam. In this case, the waist is located at the flat exit face of the fiber, with a waist diameter approximately 1.2 to 1.5 times the core diameter. If the core diameter is 6 μm and λ = 0.7 μm, Equation 4.20 gives a divergence half-angle of about 3.2°. Again, this can be reduced by a collimating lens.

4.5 SCATTERING FROM PARTICLES

Small dielectric particles suspended in an aerosol or in a liquid will scatter electromagnetic waves in a manner that, as seen in several instances earlier, depends on the ratio of particle size to wavelength. For particles that will stay suspended for a long time in an aerosol or liquid solution, the particle sizes are very small—on the order of nanometers to micrometers. Thus, typical sizes of suspended particles are often smaller than the wavelength of visible light, but sometimes they can be comparable in size to the wavelength or larger. The reason scattering is discussed in this chapter (even though the wavelength is not much smaller than the particles) is that most scattering of interest involves optical waves.

The mechanism for the scattering of electromagnetic waves from particles is similar to that in Section 1.6, which describes the interaction between **E** fields and dielectric materials. When an incident wave passes through a particle, the **E** field causes the electric dipoles in the particle's material (either induced or already existing) to align and alternate with the field, or, in conducting particles, causes free electrons to oscillate back and forth at the same frequency as the incident field. These oscillating charges act as small antennas (see Section 3.7), reradiating a wave that becomes the scattered wave.

The pattern of the scattered wave from this particle depends on the relative phases of the wavelets emanating from the various portions of the particle. Thus, the pattern is sensitive to the size and shape of the particle. If the particle is very small compared with a wavelength, its radiation pattern falls into the classification of *Rayleigh* scattering. If its size is on the same order as a wavelength, the pattern is much more complex and the scattering is known as *Mie* scattering. The characteristics of these two scattering regimes are discussed in more detail in the following sections.

Of course, there are many particles in the scattering cloud, so the individual waves from each particle combine to form the entire scattered wave. In most cases of interest, the individual particles are randomly located in the cloud, so the waves from these particles have random phases uniformly distributed over 0 to 360° when they reach the observation point. When their **E** fields add, the resultant total **E** field has a magnitude whose average is statistically equal to the square root of the sum of all the individual **E**-field magnitudes. The power density in the scattered wave, proportional to the square of the resultant **E**-field amplitude, is therefore equal to the sum of the power density scattered from each particle. This is an example of the *incoherent* addition of powers from individual particles. If there are N particles in the cloud and each particle scatters P power, the total average power in the scattered wave is NP.

4.5.1 RAYLEIGH SCATTERING

When the particle is small compared to a wavelength, the scattering contributions coming from each segment of the particle are approximately in phase. Thus the particle acts as a single small dipole antenna. Section 3.7 shows that the radiation pattern from a small dipole is uniform in angle in the plane perpendicular to the **E** field, radiating equally in all directions in that plane, but falls off in the direction parallel to the **E**-field vector in the plane containing **E** (as shown in Figure 3.51 earlier). The Rayleigh scattering pattern follows that same doughnut-shaped behavior, as indicated in Figure 4.19: It scatters uniformly forward, sideways, and backward, decreasing only in the direction aligned with the incident electric field.

The magnitude of the scattering from a Rayleigh particle depends strongly—in fact to the fourth power—on the size of the particle compared with the wavelength. If the effective particle size is s, the power-scattering efficiency of the particle is proportional to $(s/\lambda)^4$. Over the visible wavelengths, there is a dramatic change in the scattering power for a particle of a given size when going from the short-wavelength end of the spectrum to the long-wavelength end. Figure 4.20 shows that the relative scattering efficiency is more than nine times larger for blue light than for red light. This helps explain the blue color of the sky. We see scattered sunlight when we look up through the atmosphere, and scattering by the molecules in the air is much more effective for the blue portion of sunlight than for red. Even though the scattering from each air molecule is very small, the huge number of molecules makes the total scattered power visible. Random fluctuations in the air density also cause scattering with the same behavior.

The $(s/\lambda)^4$ scattering dependence that is characteristic of Rayleigh scattering also applies for a fixed wavelength as the particle size varies. Figure 4.21 shows the very large variation in relative scattering efficiency for a fixed wavelength as the particle size varies over just a tenfold range. Obviously, larger particles are much more efficient light scatterers than small particles in the Rayleigh regime.

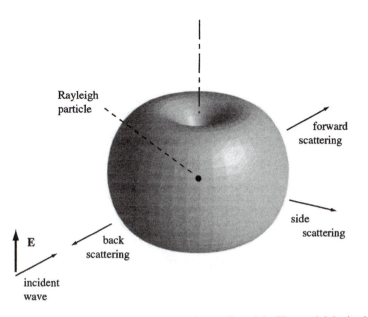

FIGURE 4.19 A polar plot of the scattering efficiency of a small particle. The particle's size is much smaller than the wavelength of the incident light, so its scattering behavior follows Rayleigh scattering equations. Note that scattering is uniform in the plane perpendicular to the incident **E**-field vector, but it falls to zero in the direction parallel to the **E** field. The polar plot therefore has a doughnut shape.

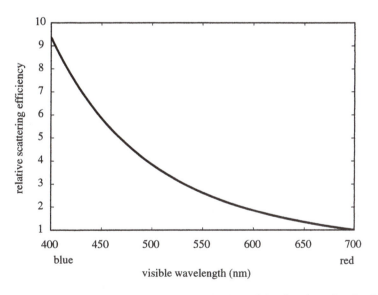

FIGURE 4.20 The relative scattering efficiency of a Rayleigh particle of a given size for different visible wavelengths. Due to the fourth-power wavelength dependence, blue light is scattered much more than red light.

4.5.2 MIE SCATTERING

For larger particles, ones whose sizes are on the order of the wavelength of light, the scattering pattern and scattering efficiency becomes much more complicated than the rather uniform pattern of the Rayleigh particle. Because the contributions to the scattered wave emanating from different parts of the particle are spread over distances that are a significant fraction of a wavelength (or

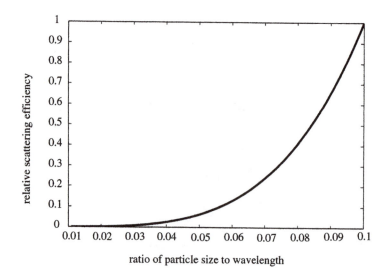

FIGURE 4.21 The relative scattering efficiency of Rayleigh-sized particles of varying sizes as a ratio to wavelength. The fourth-power dependence that is characteristic of Rayleigh scattering makes larger particles scatter considerably more efficiently than smaller particles.

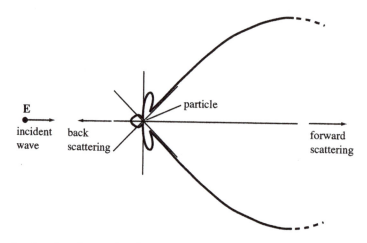

FIGURE 4.22 A polar plot of scattering from a Mie-sized spherical particle. This plot shows scattering efficiency as a function of angle in the plane perpendicular to the incident **E** field. In this example, the particle's diameter is 1.27 times the wavelength and the particle's refractive index is 1.25. Note the large forward-scattering component characteristic of Mie scattering as opposed to the uniform scattering expected in this plane for much smaller Rayleigh particles.

even a few wavelengths) apart, the large phase variations of these contributions cause major constructive and destructive interference that is a sensitive function of the angle, shape, orientation, refractive index, and conductivity of the particle. Thus the pattern of Mie scattering can be very irregular, with numerous peaks and valleys at various angles. For example, Figure 4.22 shows a polar plot of the Mie scattering in the plane perpendicular to the incident **E** field for a spherical particle that is 1.27 wavelengths in diameter with a refractive index of 1.25. Even this simple spherically shaped particle displays an irregular scattering pattern.

   Although the Mie patterns are relatively complex, there is one characteristic that is commonly seen in the patterns from spherical and similarly shaped particles. The forward-scattered power, which is the scattering into a cone in the same direction as the incident wave, is greater than the scattered power in other directions (this is known as the Mie effect). The forward-scattering component becomes even more pronounced as the particle diameter increases.

You can easily demonstrate these effects in the lab or at home by passing a light beam (from a laser pointer or a flashlight, for example) through a solution of scattering particles such as a glass of milk that has been diluted amply with water so the beam passes through several centimeters without suffering too much attenuation. In a darkened room, observe the brightness of the scattering as a function of angle (but be careful not to look directly into the transmitted laser beam) to see the increase in scattering in the forward direction compared with the side and back directions.

If you use the white beam from a flashlight, notice also that the color of the forward-scattered light takes on a reddish or yellowish tint. This is due to the higher amount of scattering of the blue light out of the way than of the red light, for the reason mentioned above. (This is also the source of beautiful red sunsets, accentuated when there is an excess of haze or pollution in the air.) If you are using a polarized laser, notice that the scattering off to the side in the direction aligned with the incident **E** field is lower than that in the perpendicular plane, as evident in Figure 4.19 for Rayleigh particles. This characteristic is seen in smaller-sized Mie particles as well as Rayleigh particles.

When the particle size gets very large (much larger than the wavelength of the light), geometrical optics becomes the applicable analysis tool and ray tracing can be used, as discussed in the first part of this chapter.

The increase in both Rayleigh and Mie scattering power when the particle size gets larger sometimes has unfortunate consequences in human vision as a person gets older. With aging (and exposure to ultraviolet rays), some people will develop cataracts in the lenses of their eyes. These cataracts are caused by aggregation of proteins in the lens, producing density variations with corresponding refractive index variations. These result in small scattering centers. As the cataracts grow, they scatter more light out of the normal path to the retina, resulting in dimmer and blurred images. When severe enough, the cataracts have to be surgically removed to restore reasonable vision. However, even before they cause noticeably blurred images, developing cataracts will cause scattering. This is especially evident as "halos" around a bright light source (forward scattering) that can obscure the images of nearby objects. Many older people complain of this halo effect when driving at night in the presence of oncoming headlights.

4.6 PHOTON INTERACTIONS WITH TISSUES

It is obvious by visual inspection that the tissues of the body have much different optical properties than typical dielectric materials used in optics, such as glass. For example, consider what happens when a bright beam of light (from a flashlight or laser) is shone through your closed fingers and observed from the opposite side in a darkened room. Even though the beam may be fairly directed (collimated) when entering the tissue, by the time it exits it has spread into a large glow. It also has lost some of its intensity by absorption. This illustrates two main characteristics of the optical properties of tissues (as represented here by soft tissue): First, there is a large amount of scattering by the microstructure of the tissue. Second, there is a fair amount of absorption, which in many tissues is wavelength-dependent and which therefore imparts a color to the tissue. We cover these aspects in more detail in the next two sections.

4.6.1 LIGHT SCATTERING IN TISSUES AND PHOTON MIGRATION

A simplified picture of how light propagates through tissue is offered in Figure 4.23. This shows the paths that a light beam might take as it passes through the tissue. The most obvious feature is the high degree of multiple scattering that occurs as the light encounters numerous layers of inhomogeneous tissue components and multiple sites of scattering. The multiple scattering is indicated by the zigzag path of the light rays. Upon each scattering event, the direction of the light is scrambled.

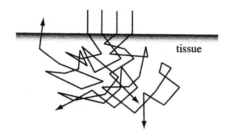

FIGURE 4.23   A simple picture showing the paths that photons might take in traveling through soft tissue. Note the high degree of multiple scattering, making imaging with light difficult at any depth beneath the skin's surface.

The use of rays here to describe the light propagation is not strictly valid but is used as a visualization tool. An alternative description is to consider the paths that photons (the quantum-mechanical particles that make up the energy of a light beam) would take as they transit through the tissue. The paths may look similar to the zigzag paths of Figure 4.23. This viewpoint, known as a study of *photon migration* in tissue, is a rich research topic. Statistical estimates of the propagation of photons through various types of tissue can be made from this viewpoint. Many of these studies use the so-called Monte Carlo computer technique, where a vast number of individual photons are tracked one at a time through the tissue, each one undergoing a large number of random scattering events, then the paths are added up to arrive at an estimate of the total effect on the light beam.

An estimate of the degree of the multiple scattering can be obtained from the value of the scattering coefficient μ_s' of the tissue. For typical soft tissue, μ_s' is approximately in the range 0.5 to 4 mm^{-1}. In rough terms, this means that a photon will travel only a distance of $1/\mu_s' = 0.25$ to 2 mm before encountering the next scattering event. Even in a small volume of tissue, there are many scattering events scrambling the path of the light.

The high degree of multiple scattering in tissue makes ordinary optical microscopy difficult at any depth below the surface of the skin. It is like trying to see objects through a very dense fog. There is, however, a new development in tissue microscopy, called optical coherence tomography or OCT, which uses the partial temporal coherence properties of nonlaser sources to image objects at moderate distances (a few millimeters) beneath the surface of the skin.

4.6.2   Tissue Absorption and Spectroscopy

In addition to being highly scattering, typical tissues (other than the humor of the eye) have a moderate amount of absorption. The magnitude of tissue absorption may be estimated from the absorption coefficient μ_a, which is approximately 0.01 to 1 mm^{-1} for soft tissues (there is a large amount of variation between tissue types and with wavelength). This means a light beam will travel approximately $1/\mu_a = 1$ to 100 mm before losing an appreciable amount of its energy by absorption. Note that the absorption coefficient is smaller than the scattering coefficient. That means that a photon on average will encounter many scattering events before being absorbed or exiting out from the tissue.

One interesting use of optical absorption in tissues is for diagnostic purposes. Here the wavelength dependence of the absorption is used to measure the state of the tissues, either for detecting a disease condition or for monitoring the local environment of the tissue. This is using *spectroscopy* for diagnostics or sensing. For example, it is well known that when blood is oxygenated, it has a red color; when the blood oxygen is depleted, it takes on a blue color. In reflected light, arteries look reddish and veins look bluish. The reason for this is that oxygen is carried predominantly by hemoglobin molecules found in red blood cells. When hemoglobin is oxygenated (oxyhemoglobin, HbO_2), it absorbs red light to a lesser degree than when it has lost oxygen (reduced to hemoglobin, Hb).

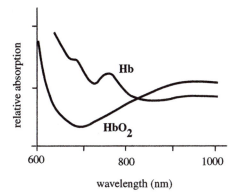

wavelength (nm)

FIGURE 4.24   The absorption characteristics of oxyhemoglobin (HbO_2) and hemoglobin (Hb) as a function of wavelength. Oxyhemoglobin absorbs less red light than hemoglobin, so oxygenated blood looks redder than deoxygenated blood. This effect is used in pulse oximeters, which use red light to noninvasively measure the oxygen saturation of a patient. A second (or more) wavelength at the isosbestic point—where absorption is not sensitive to oxygen percentage, near 805 nm—is often employed to compensate for other optical variables.

This characteristic is shown in Figure 4.24, which is the absorption curve for both states of hemoglobin as a function of wavelength. Note that at a red color (say $\lambda = 660$ nm), the absorption is less for oxyhemoglobin than for deoxygenated hemoglobin. Thus red light from an LED passing through perfused tissue will undergo a variable amount of absorption depending upon the degree of oxygenation of the blood. This allows the measurement of the oxygen saturation of the blood with relatively simple devices known as pulse oximeters, which clamp on the finger, toe, or ear lobe. In-dwelling fiber-optic oximeters also have been developed that can be inserted directly into an artery. Usually two or more wavelengths of light are used to account for the variability in tissue other than that caused by the concentration of oxygen. For example, Figure 4.24 shows that at a wavelength of about 805 nm, absorption is relatively unaffected by the degree of oxygenation; this is an *isosbestic* point. The ratio of absorption at these two wavelengths, 660 and 805 nm, will remain sensitive to oxygenation while being less sensitive to other factors.

There are other spectroscopic uses of light for monitoring the state of tissues in the body. Several of these are currently being investigated for their clinical usefulness. Fluorescence induced in various tissues (autofluorescence) by an external light source such as a laser can yield information about the nature of the tissue, such as discriminating calcified plaque from soft plaque inside arteries. Optical fibers carry the laser light to the tissue and collect the emitted fluorescence. Raman scattering, which is very specific to the tissue type but also very weak in signal strength, is being investigated for diagnostic applications as well.

5 Dosimetry

5.1 INTRODUCTION

Dosimetry consists of two parts. The first part is the determination of the *incident fields*, which are produced by some kind of source. These incident fields are either measured (with no object present) or calculated from a knowledge of the source. The second part is the determination of the **E** and **B** fields inside an object exposed to the incident fields. The fields inside an object are called the *internal fields*. The internal fields are also either measured or calculated.

Sometimes internal fields are measured in experimental animals, and sometimes they are measured in models consisting of material that has permittivity and conductivity similar to that of animal tissue. These models are sometimes called *phantoms*. Because measurements of internal fields in humans cannot be made, measurements in phantoms of humans are made to determine what the internal fields would be in the human body. When internal fields are calculated, various mathematical models are used to represent humans and other animals, as explained below. In bioelectromagnetics, information about the internal fields is usually desired so that effects of the internal fields on the biological system can be determined.

Dosimetry can be divided into two categories: *macroscopic* and *microscopic* dosimetry. In macroscopic dosimetry, the EM fields are determined as an average over some small volume of space, such as in mathematical cells that are centimeters or millimeters in size. For example, if the mathematical cell size is 1 mm on a side, then the **E** field in a given mathematical cell is assumed to have the same value everywhere within the 1 mm^3 volume of that cell. In other words, the **E** field is averaged over the volume of the cell. The **B** field is also averaged over the cell. These are called macroscopic EM fields. In contrast, in microscopic dosimetry, the EM fields are determined at a microscopic level, such as the cellular level in biological systems. Or, equivalently, the mathematical cells over which the EM fields are determined are microscopic in size.

Historically, much more has been done in macroscopic dosimetry than in microscopic dosimetry. Only recently has much work been done in microscopic dosimetry. One technique is first to determine the macroscopic fields, then "zoom in" to find the fields on a microscopic level. Microscopic dosimetry is needed to learn more about how EM fields interact with biological systems at the cellular level, but both calculations and measurements are much more difficult for microscopic dosimetry than for macroscopic dosimetry. One obvious difficulty in microscopic dosimetry is managing the huge amount of data involved in systems that consist of millions of biological cells.

This chapter discusses the principles and ideas involved in dosimetry in two cases: when the wavelength is large compared with the object (see Chapter 2) and when the wavelength is about the same size as the object (see Chapter 3). Dosimetry is not discussed when the wavelength is very small compared to the size of the object because in that case, the internal fields are confined to a very thin region near the surface of the object. Only the dosimetry of objects in free space is discussed in this chapter. The principles and characteristic behaviors related to *in vitro* dosimetry can be inferred from the discussions of internal **E** fields in Chapters 2 and 3, taking into account that SARs are proportional to the square of the internal **E** fields.

Dosimetry is a complicated subject, and the literature describing the development and implementation of both theoretical and experimental dosimetric techniques and the resulting dosimetric data is extensive. The purpose of this chapter is not to give a comprehensive review or discussion of dosimetric techniques or to give a comprehensive set of data for the internal fields for various models of humans and other animals. Instead, it is to help you understand the elementary ideas

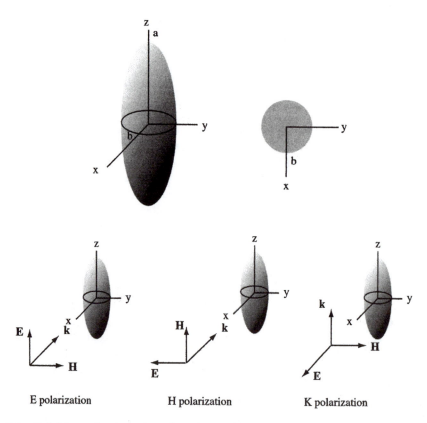

FIGURE 5.1 Definitions of polarizations for a body of rotation about the z axis. For convenience, the polarizations are illustrated with respect to a prolate spheroid, but they apply to any body of rotation. (Adapted from Figure 3.37, Durney, C. H., Massoudi, H., and Iskander, M. F., *Radiofrequency Radiation Dosimetry Handbook*, 4th edition, Report USAFSAM-TR-85-73, USAF School of Aerospace Medicine, Aerospace Medical Division (AFSC), Brooks Air Force Base, TX 78235-5301, 1986.)

involved in dosimetry and to provide a brief introduction to some of the techniques used in dosimetry. To do so, elementary results from some of the early work with simple models, primarily as summarized in the fourth edition of the *Radiofrequency Radiation Dosimetry Handbook*, are used as examples.

5.2 SOME DEFINITIONS AND PARAMETERS USED IN DOSIMETRY

This section provides definitions of polarizations and descriptions of the electrical properties of the human body, both of which are needed for subsequent discussions of dosimetry.

5.2.1 DEFINITIONS OF POLARIZATIONS

The calculated **E** fields inside prolate spheroidal models in Section 2.3 illustrate the general characteristic that internal fields vary with the orientation of the incident fields with respect to the object. The orientation of the incident **E** field with respect to the object is called *polarization*. For objects of rotation (those with circular symmetry about the long axis), three polarizations are defined: E, H, and K, as illustrated in terms of a prolate spheroidal model in Figure 5.1. E polarization is when the incident **E** field lies along the axis of the object, H polarization is when the incident **H** field lies along the long axis, and K polarization is when the propagation vector **k** lies along the long axis of the object.

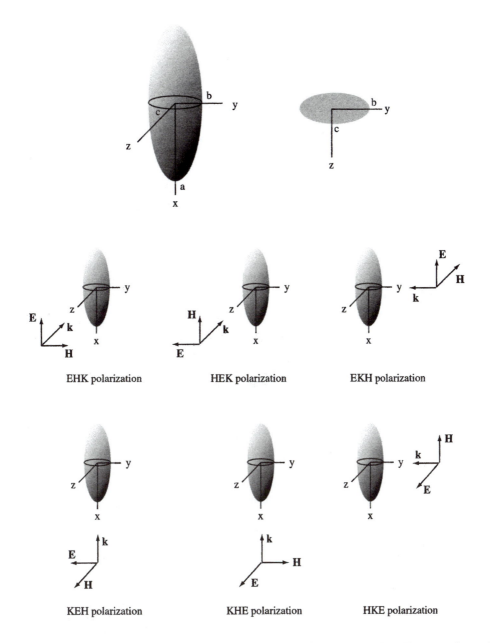

FIGURE 5.2 Definitions of polarizations for a body that is not a body of rotation. For convenience, the polarizations are illustrated with respect to an ellipsoid, but they apply to other objects as well. (Adapted from Figure 3.38, Durney, C. H., Massoudi, H., and Iskander, M. F., *Radiofrequency Radiation Dosimetry Handbook*, 4th edition, Report USAFSAM-TR-85-73, USAF School of Aerospace Medicine, Aerospace Medical Division (AFSC), Brooks Air Force Base, TX 78235-5301, 1986.)

For objects that are not objects of rotation, such as the human body, six polarizations are defined, as illustrated in Figure 5.2 in terms of an ellipsoid. An ellipsoid has three semiaxes; the lengths are labeled as a, b, and c in Figure 5.2, with $a > b > c$, and a lies along the x axis, b along the y axis, and c along the z axis. The polarizations are defined with respect to which of the vectors **E**, **H**, or **k** lie along which of the three semiaxes. For example, in EHK polarization, **E** lies along a, **H** along b, and **k** along c.

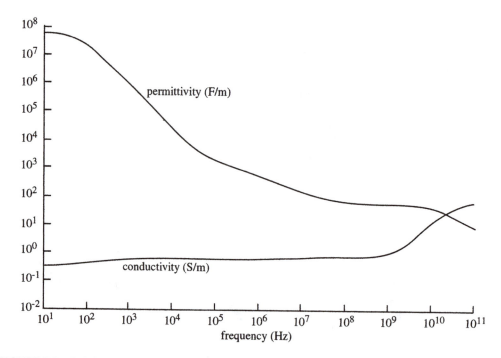

FIGURE 5.3   Relative permittivity and effective conductivity of muscle tissue (fibers parallel to the incident **E**) as a function of frequency. (Adapted from Figure C29, Gabriel, C., Compilation of the Dielectric Properties of Body Tissues at RF and Microwave Frequencies, Report AL/OE-TR-1996-0037, Occupational and Environmental Health Directorate Radiofrequency Radiation Division, Brooks AFB, TX 78235-5102, 1996.)

5.2.2   ELECTRICAL PROPERTIES OF THE HUMAN BODY

Both theoretical and experimental dosimetry require a knowledge of the electrical properties of the object for which dosimetry is being assessed. In particular, when the object is the human body, its electrical properties must be known to calculate internal fields or to construct phantoms on which measurements can be made. The electrical properties of the human body are usually specified either in terms of relative permittivity and effective conductivity or in terms of complex relative permittivity (see Sections 1.6 and 1.7). In general, the relative permittivity and effective conductivity of body tissues are a strong function of frequency. Each tissue in the body has a different variation with frequency. All of this must be taken into account in dosimetry.

As an example, Figure 5.3 shows the relative permittivity and effective conductivity of muscle tissue (fibers parallel to the incident electric field) as a function of frequency from 10 Hz to 100 GHz. The relative permittivity changes about seven orders of magnitude over that range, a wide variation, indeed. In contrast, the effective conductivity changes only about two orders of magnitude, being relatively flat with frequency up to about 1 GHz. The average of relative permittivity and of effective conductivity of all the tissues in the human body is equal to about two-thirds that of muscle tissue. Consequently, in simple homogeneous models of the human body (like prolate spheroids) used in dosimetry calculations, the relative permittivity and effective conductivity are often taken to be two-thirds that of muscle.

The relative permittivity and effective conductivity of fat tissue are shown in Figure 5.4. Both parameters are about ten times lower for fat than for muscle. Similarly, other body permittivities and conductivities vary widely, depending on the tissue type. This difference in properties is a significant factor in many applications involving internal EM fields as explained in previous chapters and again in Chapter 6.

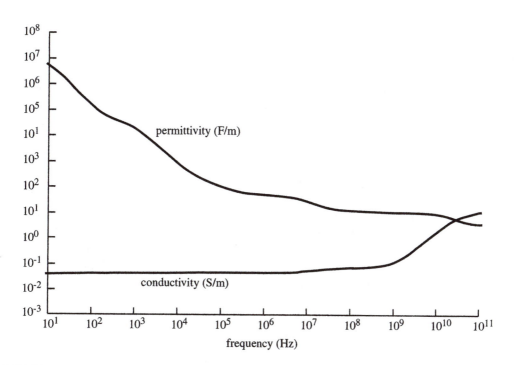

FIGURE 5.4 Relative permittivity and effective conductivity of fat tissue as a function of frequency. (Adapted from Figure C17, Gabriel, C., Compilation of the Dielectric Properties of Body Tissues at RF and Microwave Frequencies, Report AL/OE-TR-1996-0037, Occupational and Environmental Health Directorate Radiofrequency Radiation Division, Brooks AFB, TX 78235-5102, 1996.)

5.3 ENERGY ABSORPTION (SAR)

As explained in Section 1.15, the penetration of incident EM fields into biological bodies decreases as frequency increases. The general effect is illustrated in Figure 1.29 by the strong decrease of skin depth as frequency increases. But because Figure 1.29 is for a dielectric halfspace, it does not show other effects that are related to the size of the object. The energy absorbed by an object exposed to incident EM fields is a function of frequency, and of the size, shape, and electrical properties of the object. This section discusses the characteristics of energy absorption in terms of the SAR (see Section 1.7), first at low frequencies where the wavelength is long compared with the object size and then at higher frequencies where resonance effects can occur.

5.3.1 SARs at Low Frequencies

As explained in Section 2.2, the **E** and **B** fields are approximately uncoupled at low frequencies, that is, at frequencies low enough that the wavelength is large compared with the size of the object. In this frequency range, then, dosimetry consists of determining the internal fields due to the incident **E** field acting alone and then due to the incident **B** field acting alone, as illustrated in Figure 2.1.

In measuring or calculating the internal fields at low frequencies, various models are used to represent humans or other animals. In early work, spherical models were used. Spheres obviously do not represent the shape of the animals very well, but much useful information that served as a basis for calculations in more realistic models was obtained from spherical models. Subsequently, spheroidal (egg-shaped) and ellipsoidal models were used to represent animal shapes more realistically. Spherical, spheroidal, and ellipsoidal models were particularly useful because analytical, or closed-form, solutions could be obtained for them at low frequencies. That is, Maxwell's equations could be solved and mathematical expressions for the internal **E** and **H** fields could be obtained. Such solutions provided valuable understanding about the characteristics of internal fields.

Later, other models with more realistic shapes were used in both experimental measurements and in calculations. For experimental measurements, figurines were used. For calculations, so-called *block models* were used. These block models consist of cubical mathematical cells arranged to approximate the shape of human and other animal bodies. Analytical solutions cannot be obtained for these models. Instead, *numerical methods* are used to calculate the internal fields. These numerical methods consist of solving Maxwell's equations using some kind of computer technique that gives the **E** and **H** fields in each mathematical cell of the model. In some of these numerical techniques, cubical mathematical cells are used; in others, pyramidal cells are used.

Some commonly used numerical methods are the moment method, the finite-element method, finite-difference time-domain (FDTD) method, finite-difference frequency-domain (FDFD) method, and impedance method. In general, models with more realistic shapes require a larger number of smaller mathematical cells. With a larger number of smaller mathematical cells the fields can be calculated with finer resolution, but this also requires more computer memory and computational time. In recent years, computers have become more powerful, allowing more sophisticated dosimetry calculations. Calculating fields with more resolution is not enough, however. Having huge data files consisting of **E** and **H** fields in each of many mathematical cells does not necessarily provide insight into the characteristic behaviors of these fields. An understanding of this characteristic behavior is important in interpreting and evaluating the interactions of EM fields with biological systems.

The nature of the internal fields at very low frequencies is adequately illustrated by the calculation of the internal **E** fields in two very simple cases: a prolate spheroid exposed to an incident **E** field of 1 kV/m, which is typical of environmental fields, and a prolate spheroid exposed to an incident 60-Hz **B** field of 1 mT, which is typical of that of a hair dryer. These are the same as the examples illustrated in Figures 2.6 and 2.31. The prolate spheroid in each case is approximately the size of an average man. The conductivity, which dominates over the permittivity in determining the internal **E** at low frequencies, is 0.067 S/m, which is about two-thirds that of muscle tissue at 60 Hz.

One important consideration related to dosimetry is heating of tissue that might be caused by the internal **E** fields. To consider possible heating effects at low frequencies, first calculate from the SAR the temperature rise that would be produced by an internal **E** field of 1 V/m. Then calculate the temperature rise for any internal **E** field by multiplying the result by the square of that **E**, since the SAR varies as E^2. According to Equation 1.12, the SAR in the prolate spheroids for the above examples is given by SAR $= \sigma_{eff} E^2/2\rho = 0.067 \times 1^2/2000 = 0.0335 \times 10^{-3}$ W/kg if we assume the mass density of tissue is about the same as that of water, which is 1000 kg/m³. The power transferred to one gram of tissue by the **E** would be $0.0335 \times 10^{-3} \times 10^{-3} = 0.0335 \times 10^{-6}$ W. The one gram of tissue would therefore absorb 0.0335×10^{-6} joules of energy in one second, since energy is equal to power × time. Since 4.186 joules are required to raise one gram of tissue 1°C, the temperature rise of the tissue would be $0.0335 \times 10^{-6}/4.186 = 8.00 \times 10^{-9}$ °C if all the absorbed energy were transformed into heat (and heat diffusion is ignored).

For the internal **E** fields in Figure 2.6, the temperature rise calculated above for an internal **E** of 1 V/m would be multiplied by the square of the internal **E**. Thus for the largest internal **E** of Figure 2.6 of 260 μV/m, the temperature rise would be $8.00 \times 10^{-9} \times (260 \times 10^{-6})^2 = 5.41 \times 10^{-16}$ °C. This is obviously a negligible rise in temperature. Even for the much larger internal **E** of 51 mV/m produced by the incident **B** of Figure 2.31, the temperature rise would be only 2.08×10^{-11} °C. Although these results are for a very simple model, they are consistent with the more general results that heating caused by typical low-frequency incident **E** and **B** fields is negligible.

Comparison of these calculated internal **E** fields with endogenous fields in biological systems also provides some perspective. Typical **E** fields across cell membranes are about 10^7 V/m. The threshold for nerve stimulation is typically about 6.2 V/m. Thus internal fields of μV/m or even

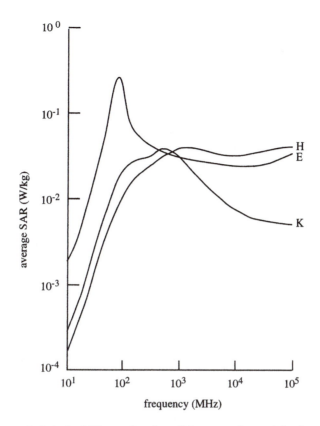

FIGURE 5.5 Average whole-body SAR as a function of frequency for models of an average man in free space for three polarizations, E, H, and K. The incident wave is a planewave with a power density of 1 mW/cm². (Adapted from Figure 3.39, Durney, C. H., Massoudi, H., and Iskander, M. F., *Radiofrequency Radiation Dosimetry Handbook*, 4th edition, Report USAFSAM-TR-85-73, USAF School of Aerospace Medicine, Aerospace Medical Division (AFSC), Brooks Air Force Base, TX 78235-5301, 1986.)

mV/m are small compared with typical endogenous fields. On the other hand, low-frequency incident **E** fields can produce shocks and burns. Because **E** fields at the surface could be much higher than internal **E** fields, low-frequency **E** fields might produce biological effects related to interactions at the surface.

5.3.2 SAR as a Function of Frequency

The general characteristics of the average whole-body SAR as a function of frequency for a model of an average man irradiated by an incident planewave with a power density of 1 mW/cm² (see Poynting vector in Section 3.4.3) are shown in Figure 5.5. The calculated results shown in the figure are the results of early work using a combination of simple models (prolate spheroid, cylinder, capped cylinder), empirical techniques, and for part of the graph, interpolated estimations. Several methods of calculation were used over various parts of the frequency range. At low frequencies, a long-wavelength approximation was made. The extended-boundary-condition method (EBCM) was used up to approximately the resonant frequency (see Section 3.6). Above that, the iterative EBCM (IEBCM) method was used. Other methods include the classical solution to Maxwell's equations for cylinders and the surface integral equation (SIE) method.

Although more sophisticated methods can now be used because computing power has increased so much since these calculations were made, these early results are useful because they illustrate the elementary features of the SAR variation with frequency. They also illustrate the methods that were first used to understand the basic characterisitics of SARs for humans and other animals. Moment-method frequency-domain calculations in block models have provided much useful dosimetry information. FDFD methods have proven to be very powerful for calculating internal EM fields. Finite-element methods and finite-difference frequency-domain (FDFD) methods have also been used in electromagnetic dosimetry calculations. The literature contains extensive information about dosimetry methods and calculations, but further details are much beyond the scope of this book.

For all three polarizations, the SAR varies approximately as the square of the frequency at low frequencies. For E polarization, a resonance (see Section 3.6) occurs at about 80 MHz. Compared with the cavity resonance discussed in Section 3.6, the resonance shown in Figure 5.5 has a very low Q, which is due primarily to the much lower conductivity of the biological body. For long thin metallic objects, such as a wire antenna, a resonance occurs when the length of the object is about equal to a half-wavelength. For biological objects, which are generally thicker and of lower conductivity, the resonance occurs when the object length is about four-tenths of a wavelength. At frequencies above resonance, the SAR varies approximately as the inverse of the frequency.

At frequencies below resonance, the SAR for E polarization is highest, for H polarization it is lowest, and for K polarization it is in between the other two. Qualitative explanations of this effect are given in Section 5.4.

To illustrate how the SAR frequency dependence varies with object size, Figure 5.6 shows the average whole-body SAR for a model of a medium-sized rat. The resonant frequency for E polarization in this case is about 600 MHz, considerably higher than for the average man. This is to be expected because the rat is much shorter than the man. Again, resonance ocurs when the object is about four-tenths of a wavelength long. The resonance in the rat is less pronounced than in the man, probably because the man is relatively thinner than the rat. For the rat, the SAR also varies approximately as the frequency squared below resonance and as the inverse of the frequency above resonance.

Calculations in models with more realistic shapes show additional bumps on the average whole-body SAR graph that are caused by local resonance effects of the head, arms, and legs. The overall shape of the SAR graph is basically the same, however, as that obtained for simpler models. Inhomogeneous models have also been used to simulate the presence of organs and other details of the body. Calculations in inhomogeneous models show that the differing permittivities and conductivities of the various tissues of the body can cause the SAR to vary over the body. This local variation can also be a strong function of frequency. Even in homogeneous models, the SAR can vary significantly over the body, as illustrated in Section 3.4. In some cases, areas of intense local SARs can occur. These are sometimes called "hotspots," which is not precise terminology because "hot" refers to temperature, but temperature inside the body depends not only on the absorbed energy but also on the thermal properties of the body.

5.4 EFFECTS OF POLARIZATION ON SAR

Figures 5.5 and 5.6 show that the SARs for both man-sized and rat-sized models vary significantly with polarization. Not only in these two cases, but also in general, polarization has a strong effect on SARs. This effect can be explained in terms of two general behaviors described in Sections 2.3 and 2.5 in connection with Figures 2.6 and 2.31. These general behaviors are (1) the internal $\mathbf{E}$ field is generally greater when the $\mathbf{E}_{inc}$ is "mostly parallel" to the body surface than when it is "mostly normal" to the body surface, and (2) the internal $\mathbf{E}$ is generally greater when the cross-sectional area intercepted by the $\mathbf{H}_{inc}$ is greater than it is when the intercepted cross-sectional area is smaller. (Sometimes we use $\mathbf{B}$ and $\mathbf{H}$ almost interchangeably, since $\mathbf{B} = \mu\mathbf{H}$ and for biological systems the permeability μ is approximately equal to μ_0, that of free space.)

These explanations are based on the low-frequency concepts that the $\mathbf{E}$ and $\mathbf{H}$ are approximately uncoupled at low frequencies and that the internal $\mathbf{E}$ is the sum of the internal $\mathbf{E}$ produced by the

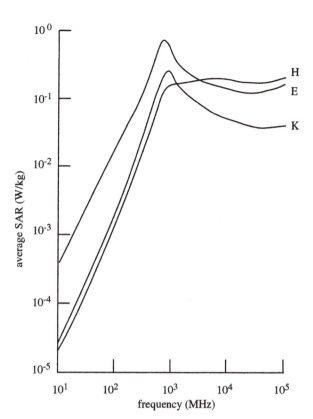

FIGURE 5.6   Average whole-body SAR as a function of frequency for models of a medium-sized rat in free space for three polarizations, E, H, and K. The incident wave is a planewave with a power density of 1 mW/cm². (Adapted from Figure 3.40, Durney, C. H., Massoudi, H., and Iskander, M. F., *Radiofrequency Radiation Dosimetry Handbook*, 4th edition, Report USAFSAM-TR-85-73, USAF School of Aerospace Medicine, Aerospace Medical Division (AFSC), Brooks Air Force Base, TX 78235-5301, 1986.)

$\mathbf{E}_{inc}$ and by the $\mathbf{H}_{inc}$. At higher frequencies, the effects are more complicated because **E** and **H** are coupled together and can strongly interact, but the ideas may have some validity even at higher frequencies. To facilitate the following discussion of how polarization affects SARs, the internal **E** field produced by $\mathbf{E}_{inc}$ is denoted as $\mathbf{E}_{Eint}$ and the internal **E** field produced by $\mathbf{H}_{inc}$ is denoted as $\mathbf{E}_{Hint}$.

Now, from Figure 5.1 we see that for E polarization, $\mathbf{E}_{inc}$ is mostly parallel to the body, and the cross-sectional area intercepted by $\mathbf{H}_{inc}$ is large compared with that of the other polarizations. Thus for E polarization, both $\mathbf{E}_{Eint}$ and $\mathbf{E}_{Hint}$ are relatively strong. For H polarization, on the other hand, $\mathbf{E}_{inc}$ is mostly normal to the body, and the cross-sectional area intercepted by $\mathbf{H}_{inc}$ is smaller than that for E polarization. Therefore, both $\mathbf{E}_{Eint}$ and $\mathbf{E}_{Hint}$ are relatively weaker than for E polarization. The SAR for E polarization is thus greater than that for H polarization. For K polarization, $\mathbf{E}_{inc}$ is mostly normal to the body, but the cross-sectional area intercepted by $\mathbf{H}_{inc}$ is large. $\mathbf{E}_{Eint}$ is therefore weak, but $\mathbf{E}_{Hint}$ is strong. The SAR for K polarization therefore is less than that for E polarization but greater than that for H polarization, as shown in Figures 5.5 and 5.6 for frequencies below resonance. These ideas are summarized in Table 5.1.

5.5   EFFECTS OF OBJECT SIZE ON SAR

Because resonance for E polarization occurs when the object length is about four-tenths of a wavelength, it is obvious that the SAR depends strongly on object size. This dependence is further illustrated in Figure 5.7, which shows SARs for an average man and a medium-sized rat for E

TABLE 5.1

Summary of Explanations for the Effects of Polarization on SARs

Polarization	E_{inc}	H_{inc}	E_{Eint}	E_{Hint}	Relative SAR
E	Mostly parallel	Intercepts large cross section	Strong	Strong	Highest
K	Mostly normal	Intercepts large cross section	Weak	Strong	Middle
H	Mostly normal	Intercepts small cross section	Weak	Weak	Lowest

polarization, both plotted on the same set of axes. The whole-body average SAR that is plotted in the figures is obtained by calculating the total energy absorbed by the object per unit time and dividing by the mass of the object. The SAR, of course, varies from point to point inside the object. Because the rat is quite different in both size and anatomical features, the spatial distribution of the SAR inside the rat is quite different from that inside the man.

Even for objects of the same basic shape but different in size, the internal SAR distribution can be quite different, depending on the frequency. For example, consider two prolate spheroids, one man-sized and one rat-sized. At 80 MHz, the internal SAR inside the man-sized spheroid would vary significantly over the volume of the spheroid. On the other hand, at 80 MHz, the internal SAR inside the rat-sized spheroid would be relatively constant. As first explained in Section 1.14, it is a matter of the size of the object compared with the wavelength. The internal SAR pattern is different in the two spheroids because the ratio of the object size to the wavelength is quite different.

On the other hand, the internal SAR distribution in the rat-sized spheroid at 600 MHz would be similar to the internal SAR distribution in the man-sized spheroid at 80 MHz, since the wavelength-to-object-size ratio is about the same in both cases. Thus, as explained in more detail in the next section, to get similar internal SAR distributions in two objects of different sizes, each object should be irradiated at a frequency for which the ratio of object size to wavelength is approximately the same.

The SAR in an object can also be affected by the presence of other objects. For example, when an object is placed on a perfectly conducting plane, the resonant frequency is approximately cut in half compared to the resonant frequency of the object in free space. Thus, for a man standing on a perfectly conducting plane and in good contact with the plane, the resonant frequency would be about 40 MHz. This effect occurs because the conducting plane has the effect of mirroring, or imaging, the man, making him appear to be twice as tall. For a man standing on the ground, which is not perfectly conducting, the resonant frequency would be lower than for free-space, but not half, as it would be for a perfectly conducting plane. Also, shoes would insulate the man from the ground, further affecting the resonant frequency.

5.6 EXTRAPOLATING FROM EXPERIMENTAL ANIMAL RESULTS TO THOSE EXPECTED IN HUMANS

Because bioelectromagnetic experiments that would require radiating people usually cannot be performed because of possible hazards, much research has been done with experimental animals to determine effects that might be expected in humans. The internal **E** fields in experimental animals exposed to specific EM fields usually differ significantly from those that would be induced in humans by the same EM fields because experimental animals differ significantly in size and shape from humans. But it is the internal EM fields, not the incident EM fields, that would cause any biological effects. Extrapolating results from experimental animals to those expected in humans must therefore be done with extreme care, and in some cases, such extrapolations may not be meaningful.

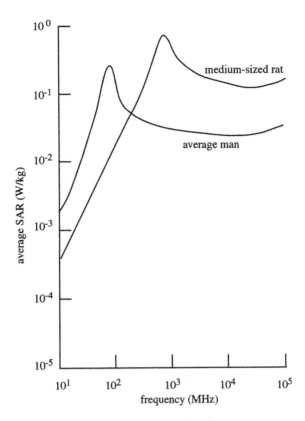

FIGURE 5.7 SARs from Figures 5.5 and 5.6 for E polarization for an average man and for a medium-sized rat plotted on the same set of axes.

For example, studying effects on people exposed to the EM fields produced by cellular telephones by studying effects on rats exposed to the same EM fields is difficult. The ideal situation would be to produce the same internal **E** and **H** field distribution in the head of a rat as that produced in the head of a human using a cellular telephone. This is not possible because the shape of the rat head is quite different from that of a human. Even to produce a similar EM pattern in the brain of a rat as that in a human brain at the same frequency is practically impossible because the brains are so different in size. The difference in the ratio of the size of the rat brain to the wavelength compared to the ratio of the size of a human brain to the wavelength would cause the internal EM fields to be very different in the two brains. If an effect in the human were caused by an internal **E** field with a given frequency and intensity acting on a given site in the brain, that would seem to be impossible to detect in experiments with rats.

On the other hand, it is possible to adjust conditions so that similarities in dosimetry between experimental animal exposure and human exposure are increased. In experiments where the biological effects are expected to be caused by heat resulting from absorbed EM energy, for example, frequencies of irradiation can be adjusted so that approximately the same whole-body SAR occurs in the experimental animals as would occur in humans. This same kind of adjustment would be appropriate for any experiment in which the biological effect is assumed to be caused by absorbed EM energy independently of the frequency.

To illustrate this kind of adjustment, consider the following situation. If an average man were exposed to a 50-MHz E-polarized planewave with a power density of 1 mW/cm^2, what radiation would produce an approximately equivalent whole-body average SAR in a medium-sized rat? Let λ_r and λ_m be the wavelengths of radiation of the rat and the man, respectively, and let h_r and h_m

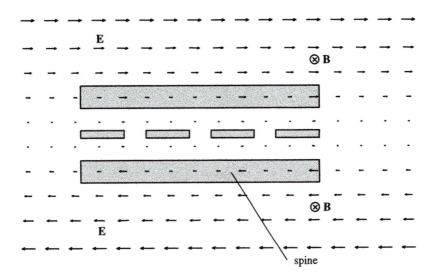

FIGURE 6.13 **E**-field pattern induced in the model without the wire present. The eddy currents follow this same pattern because current density is proportional to **E** for a homogeneous medium (muscle in this model). These results represent a reference for comparison with the results when the implant is in place. The vectors shown are interpolated from a finer grid.

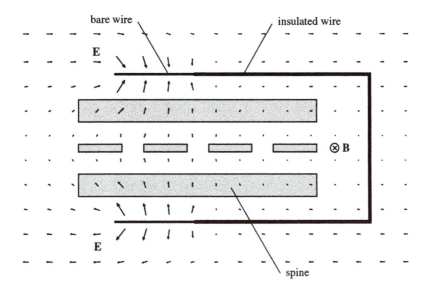

FIGURE 6.14 **E**-field pattern with U-shaped wire implant in place. Current is induced in the wire by the time-varying **B** field. The current exits one end of the wire and enters the other, causing enhanced **E** fields in the tissue near the bare ends. The vectors are interpolated from a finer grid. The **E** fields are larger than in Figure 6.13, so are plotted on a different scale.

center of circulation for the **E**-field lines near the center of the body. The **E**-field magnitude is zero there and increases toward the periphery. This behavior is typical of the eddy patterns resulting from magnetic sources, and very analogous to that seen in Figure 2.38 for a culture dish and in Figure 6.3 for an **H**-field hyperthermia applicator.

Then several cases were studied that included various configurations of the implanted wires; only two will be discussed here. The first case is for the complete U-shaped wire model (as shown in

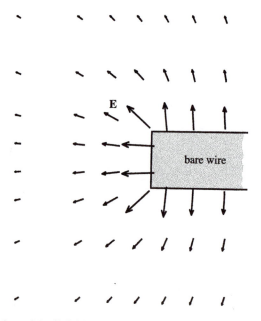

FIGURE 6.15   Close-up view of the **E** fields in Figure 6.14 near the wire ends. The fields are concentrated near the sharp corners of the wire.

Figure 6.12) with a perpendicular **B** field. Figure 6.14 shows the resulting **E**-field vectors in the plane containing the wire. The **E**-field magnitudes are larger than in the absence of the wire implant, so they are plotted to a much different scale in this figure compared with the previous figure. It is obvious that the **E** fields are modified near the bare ends of the wire. This is due to the conducting wire in the presence of the time-varying magnetic field. Current is induced to flow in the wire, much like a secondary winding in a transformer. At the low frequency of this problem (600 Hz), the current must form a complete path and close on itself. Because the wire does not form a complete loop, the current flows out of the bare wire at one end of the open loop, passes through the tissue in between, then flows back into the bare wire at the other end, completing the closed path. It must flow out the bare ends because the rest of the wire is insulated.

The **E** fields in the tissue near the bare ends of the wire are enhanced due to this current flow. This is shown in close-up view in Figure 6.15. The **E** fields are larger (more concentrated) at the small end of the wire than they are at the sides of the wire, again illustrating the concept that **E** fields concentrate around sharp boundaries of conducting objects. The magnitude of the largest **E** field in this case is about 90 times greater than at the same location without the wires present (Figure 6.13).

The current pattern inside the wire "U" is also interesting to study. This pattern is shown in Figure 6.16. As explained above, most of the current induced in the partial wire loop flows out the open ends through the tissue to complete a closed path. But, as Figure 6.16 shows, there is a *local* loop current that flows in a path contained inside the wire. This is evident by the unequal current density on the inside and outside edges of the wire. This local eddy-current pattern inside the wire is due to the finite cross-section that the wire presents to the perpendicular **B** field. If the wire were infinitely thin, there would be no local circulating current within the wire, just the global circulating current that goes through the tissue.

The second case studied was with the bottom segment of the U-shaped loop removed, leaving only the two isolated side wires. The overall **E**-field pattern is shown in Figure 6.17. The main difference here compared with the previous case is that, because the partial wire loop is now broken, there is less of a compete conducting path for the current induced in the wire. It must now flow out through tissue at both ends of both wires. This reduces the magnitude of the induced current

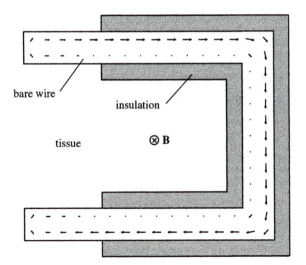

FIGURE 6.16   Current inside the wire. In addition to the global current loop indicated in Figure 6.14, there is a local loop of current inside the wire due to the finite cross section of the wire, which intercepts the perpendicular **B** field. The wire shape is not drawn to scale.

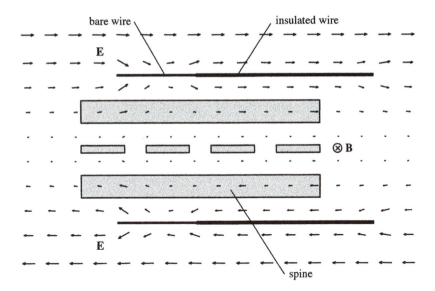

FIGURE 6.17   E-field pattern when the two side wires are disconnected from the bottom cross wire and are isolated. Less current flows in the side wires and the global current loop must now flow through tissue at both ends of the wires. The vectors shown are interpolated from a finer grid.

and correspondingly reduces the **E**-field magnitudes at the bare ends of the wires. In this case, the maximum **E**-field magnitude at the *bare* end of the wires is about 17 times that at the same location without the wires.

However, at the *other* end of the wires, the **E** field is even larger. In fact, it is the largest value seen in any of the cases studied, about 197 times the magnitude at the same location without the wires being present. This is due entirely to the configuration of the insulation at this "broken" end of the wires. As shown in Figure 6.18, it is assumed that the insulation extends all the way to the end of the wires at this end, and only the face of the wire is uninsulated and exposed to the tissue. In other words, at this end the insulation is flush with the wires. Therefore, the current that is

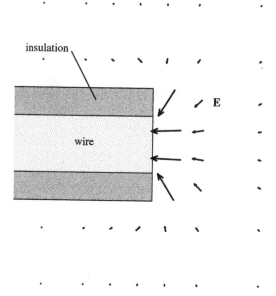

FIGURE 6.18 Close-up view of the **E** fields in Figure 6.17 near the "broken" end of each wire that is covered (except for the face) with insulation. Since the current in the wire must all flow through the small face, the current density is high here and the **E** fields are the largest for any case studied.

induced in the wires—even though smaller than before—is forced to flow entirely out the small wire ends, concentrating the current density and the **E** fields at these points. As indicated by the figure, however, the high values of **E** occur over a very small volume. Even for this worst-case scenario, it was determined that, for the assumed parameters of the problem, the **E** fields were not large enough to stimulate the nerves.

Although not all of the analyzed cases are described in this section, the ones discussed illustrate both the usefulness of one numerical technique and some of the concepts of electromagnetics covered earlier in the book.

Index